Centring Human Connections in the Education of Health Professionals

T0345259

Centring Human Connections in the Education of Health Professionals

Sherri Melrose, Caroline Park,
and Beth Perry

◊ AU PRESS

Published by AU Press, Athabasca University
1200, 10011 – 109 Street, Edmonton, AB T5J 3S8

Cover image © Kittikorn Ph. / Adobe Stock
Cover and book design by Sergiy Kozakov
Printed and bound in Canada

Library and Archives Canada Cataloguing in Publication

Centring human connections in the education of health professionals / Sherri
    Melrose, Caroline Park, and Beth Perry.

Melrose, Sherri, 1951- author. | Park, Caroline, 1948- author. | Perry, Beth, 1957-
    author.

Includes bibliographical references.

Canadiana (print) 20200310089 | Canadiana (ebook) 20200310240
    ISBN 9781771992855 (softcover) | ISBN 9781771992862 (PDF)
    ISBN 9781771992879 (HTML) | ISBN 9781771992886 (Kindle)

LCSH: Medicine—Study and teaching. | LCSH: Teacher-student relationships.

LCC R834 .M44 2020 | DDC 610.71—dc23

We acknowledge the financial support of the Government of Canada through
the Canada Book Fund (CBF) for our publishing activities and the assistance
provided by the Government of Alberta through the Alberta Media Fund.

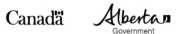

To health-care providers the world over who make a special effort to remember that each and every patient is a human being.

I think if I had to put a finger on what I consider a good education, a good radical education, it wouldn't be anything about methods or techniques. It would be loving people first.

—Myles Horton, *We Make the Road by Walking: Conversation on Education and Social Change*

Contents

Foreword

Rarely do we read a book written by educators and researchers that does not exude a technology-first mindset. Even rarer is a book that engages us in "essential human connectivity" by regularly inviting us to adopt strategies to engage and test the ideas presented through personalized examples. This is a rare book. It has a clear focus on the context of education for health professionals, yet it speaks to the essential humanness of all our interactions. So, what is essentially human? As we read chapters on culture, personalization, relationships, and the often intentionally or inadvertently hidden facets of ourselves, we get an idea of the essential human qualities and behaviours that can both support and impede teaching and learning.

This text is a scholarly work. You will find all of the claims properly referenced. You will find mention of key research ideas and authors (think Freire, Maslow, Bloom, Bandura, and others) that will be familiar to scholars of education but exciting finds to those entering scholarly study. I was pleased (and flattered of course) to see the focus on our community of inquiry (CoI) model. The CoI has been criticized for giving short shrift to the affective components of teaching and learning. This work goes a long way toward addressing that concern by showing that both social presence and cognitive presence are always mediated—and not just by technology but also by the cultural, linguistic, and affective elements of all teaching and learning contexts.

The text is also a practical work. It leverages years of the authors' scholarly research with their own experiences as long-time classroom, clinical, and online teachers—and learners! Beyond the obvious capacity to try some of the suggestions with one's own students, the reader is encouraged to test the "strategies to try" while reading. The text also provides a strong and compelling case for a variety of teacher-led interventions and learning activities that the authors have tested and refined in their own teaching.

Online education is becoming common in technology-infused classrooms, and it has often been researched and celebrated with a focus on the technical, the media, and the learning outcomes. Too often the essential humanness of the participants and activities is cloaked by the technical aspects. This book turns it all around and shows (in both theoretical and practical language) how our essential humanness affords and defines the capacity to teach and learn. With this insight, we can design and test learning activities and learning outcomes without forcing learners to park critical parts of themselves outside the technical door to learning.

This capacity to humanize is explicitly developed when confronting the curriculum—the explicit, the informal, and the hidden. The authors unpack the many influences (professional health organizations, university governance models, expectations of faculty and students) that contribute to the complex set of content and learning activities that define health education today.

Education in health care—as in other professions—evolved in the context of face-to-face interactions in training schools, universities, and health-care institutions. Now, however, professional health organizations have been hit by a tsunami of possibilities and challenges from a host of online informational, educational, and lifelong learning and networking possibilities. This is perhaps the most practical message of the book since it opens the door to real-world practice, experience, and learning by the authors as experienced teachers. There are many ways that these new tools could be used, and the book offers a great opportunity to learn from those who have been successfully teaching and actively experimenting with mediated forms of health education for years.

The final chapter is perhaps the most important. Most of us regularly think "wow, there is so much I could be doing, but where do I get the time and the motivation? I'm not a robot." Melrose, Park, and Perry do not totally resolve this challenge, but they point toward the use of humour and valuing the explicit humanness in our students, our colleagues, and most importantly ourselves. Educators, since the first use of slate boards, have been repurposing technologies to ensure that human values are celebrated and enhanced through their use. Melrose, Park, and Perry invite us to build and strengthen, and show us how to do so, our essential "human connections" within and beyond mediated learning.

Terry Anderson
Edmonton, Alberta, Canada

Centring Human Connections in the Education of Health Professionals

1

Celebrating Human Connections in Teaching

A human connection is the energy that exists between people when they feel seen, heard, and valued; when they can give and receive without judgment; and when they derive sustenance and strength from the relationship.

—Brené Brown (2010, p. 5)

The environments in which health professionals gain knowledge, skills, and attitudes that they need in their practice can be dominated by technology and mechanized procedure-oriented approaches. Health professionals achieve the competencies required by their discipline in clinical, classroom, and online settings. Health professional learners include pre-service students enrolled in higher education programs and in-service practitioners participating in graduate studies or continuing education activities. Students and practitioners in all health disciplines are expected to become, and remain, self-directed lifelong learners. Whether learners are registered in formal health profession programs or simply seek information on current best practices, they must reach out and engage with informed others and relevant resources as part of their learning.

Human connections can support learners in achieving success in all learning environments. Yet, in many instances, learners remark that they feel alone, disconnected from other students and the teacher, and bereft of human contact. Learning in isolation can negatively influence the educational experience. Learning outcomes that focus on higher-order affective domain competencies such as responding to phenomena and internalizing values are often best facilitated through human interaction and interpersonal communication.

For learners in the health professions in particular, learning in a community is essential. Health professionals provide care, kindness, and compassion to people when they are at their most vulnerable. Processes that students experience in their pre- and in-service education should model, integrate, and celebrate these human connections. Educators need to actively pursue ways to humanize the curriculum for health-care providers. In an early explanation of how educators can humanize education, Dutton (1976, p. 79) offered this simple explanation: "Make students feel ten feet tall."

In this chapter, we begin with a glimpse of what the concept of human connection means. Next, we provide a brief introduction to humanizing pedagogy with a discussion of how educational environments that embrace immediacy, praxis, and affective learning can help educators and learners to establish successful human connections. We emphasize how personalizing learning, by inviting learners to set individual goals and by offering opportunities for "voice and choice," can play a critical role in the education of health professionals. In each section, we include practical (and proven) strategies that serve one of two purposes. Some boxed strategies are designed for educators to assist them in reflecting on whether they approach learners in humanizing ways. Other boxed strategies are approaches that educators can use to help learners (in a variety of educational settings) "feel ten feet tall."

THE CONCEPT OF HUMAN CONNECTION

People engage and connect with one another in different ways and for different reasons throughout their lives. Psychologist Mathew Lieberman (2014) suggested that the human brain is wired to connect with others and that this need to connect with others is even greater than the need for food or shelter. In some instances, when connections with others extend beyond superficial conversations or interactions to include profound and meaningful communications, those involved can feel a deep sense of shared humanity.

Understanding the concept of human connection is not straightforward. The role that humanity can play in interactions is not easy to define. Most of us would associate the meaning of the word *humanity* with the simple definition of "a quality or state of being human" (Merriam-Webster, n.d.). But the definition of *humanity* also explains that the concept includes "compassionate, sympathetic or generous behaviour or disposition: the quality or state of being humane" (Merriam-Webster, n.d.). This definition is particularly important for educators who teach learners in the health professions. The definition suggests that people's behaviour toward others (e.g., educators' behaviour toward learners) is what makes them human or at least humane humans.

Deconstructing the definition further leads to a cursory examination of the requisite humanizing behaviour of compassion. *Compassion* means a "sympathetic consciousness of others' distress together with a desire to alleviate it" (Merriam-Webster, n.d.). It is beyond the scope of this book to fully explain behaviours that demonstrate compassion. However, it is important to emphasize the vital role that compassionate behaviour can play in cultivating relationships rich in humanity. Fostering human connections in health professionals' education begins when educators strive to act with compassion, to recognize distress in their students, and perhaps most notably to alleviate or reduce that distress.

In contrast, behaviours that are inhumane and lacking in compassion are not difficult to identify. Behaviours that could be described as callous, insensitive, and unfeeling are clearly inhumane. In their literature review of humane interpersonal relationships among Russian educators, Kleptsova and Balabanov (2016) noted that educators considered inhumane are likely to be more oriented to themselves, to identify others with their own ideas of good and bad, and to behave immaturely. As well, inhumane educators were described as demonstrating egoism, anger, envy, fear, cynicism, apathy, aggression, indifference, detachment, and idleness. Although educators might not intentionally act in inhumane ways, it is important to recognize that inhumane behaviours can be present and that they do not support positive, compassionate, and humane connections among educators and learners. The following strategy can initiate individual reflection and awareness building related to the importance of human connection in teaching.

What Does "Human Connection" Mean to You?

What stands out for you when you think about the concept of human connection? In your experience as a learner, can you remember a time when you felt a special connection with an educator? What role did compassion play in establishing that connection? How did this educator demonstrate humanity? Were there times when you felt stressed and overwhelmed as a learner, and at these times did this educator notice and try to help you? Document your reflections.

HUMANIZING PEDAGOGY

Immediacy

At a basic level, the word *humanizing* means making things friendlier, more understandable, and "easier for humans to relate to and appreciate" (Vocabulary.com Dictionary, n.d.). Similarly, the word *pedagogy* refers to "activities of educating or instructing; activities that impart knowledge or skill" (Vocabulary.com Dictionary, n.d.). These definitions establish that humanistic pedagogy features educational activities grounded in friendliness and relatability.

In learning environments, educators describe friendly, relatable activities as expressions of immediacy. In the 1960s, social psychologist Albert Mehrabian defined the construct of immediacy as an affective expression of emotional attachment, feelings of liking, and experiencing a sense of psychological closeness with another person (Melrose, Park, & Perry, 2013). Verbally, educators express immediacy by sharing personal examples, engaging in humour, asking questions, initiating conversations, addressing learners by name, praising learners' work, and encouraging learners to express their opinions (Gorham, 1988).

Non-verbally, immediacy is expressed by manifestations of high affect such as maintaining eye contact, leaning closer, touching, smiling, maintaining a relaxed body posture, and attending to the voice inflections of the speaker (Andersen, 1979). In higher and continuing education today, these expressions of immediacy between learners and educators continue to contribute significantly to student learning (Violanti, Kelly, Garland, & Christen, 2018).

Expressions of immediacy between educators and learners, and within learning groups, establish the foundation for humanizing pedagogy in any setting. In areas of clinical practice, new graduate nurses felt more satisfied with their jobs when their preceptors expressed immediacy by communicating an openness to their ideas and a sense of caring about their well-being (Lalonde & Hall, 2016; Quek & Shorey, 2018). In technology-rich online and blended classroom settings, higher-education nutrition students experienced a sense of closeness, community, and belonging within their class groups when educators encouraged open expression of opinions and provided opportunities for relationship building (Haar, 2018). In postgraduate e-learning classrooms, in which learners were separated geographically and temporally, nursing students highly valued interactions in which their educators acknowledged both who they were as individuals and their personal and professional responsibilities (Walkem, 2014). In staff development settings, dental hygienists were encouraged to strengthen their verbal and non-verbal immediacy skills in order to portray positivity and caring with patients (Dalonges & Fried, 2016).

Although educators might not have influence over the extent to which curricula and practice settings foster immediacy, there are always opportunities to integrate warmth and immediacy into interpersonal relationships with and among learners. The following strategy invites reflection on the construct of immediacy.

A STRATEGY TO TRY

Communicating with Immediacy

Think of your first experience in the setting where you currently teach or would like to teach. Did anyone communicate friendliness and seem to be open to getting to know you? As you reflect on those first few days in a new situation with so much to learn, how did those around you help you to feel welcome? Do you remember a particularly welcoming smile or someone who addressed you by name? Somebody who stopped what she or he was doing to listen to your question? Perhaps another person who shared a humorous anecdote or spoke with a gentle tone? Would those gestures (and how they made you feel) fit with the definition of immediacy as feeling a sense of psychological closeness to another person?

How can you affirm immediacy in your own teaching practice? Which approaches to verbal and non-verbal communication might help to reassure learners that you are open to and genuinely interested in supporting and guiding them toward success? How could you communicate this if you were teaching in an online learning milieu?

Praxis

Adult educator and philosopher Paulo Friere (1970) added to our understanding of humanizing pedagogies with his view of learners as co-creators of knowledge rather than recipients of information. Friere viewed education as a mutual process of critical consciousness in which educators and learners share a radical philosophy that actively challenges oppression, injustice, inequity, and societal conditions in the world around them. He defined this process of reflecting critically, and then acting to transform existing structures, as praxis.

In *Pedagogy of the Oppressed*, Friere (1970) argued against traditional banking approaches in which learners are perceived as empty accounts that need to be filled by educators. Banking approaches are characterized by educators who tell students what to do, what to learn, and what to think, and they seldom provide opportunities for learners to offer input, suggestions, or feedback about their education (Salazar, 2013).

In contrast, Friere (1970) called for educators to consider learners' unique abilities, backgrounds, languages, and interests rather than treating all learners the same. Known for his work to empower oppressed adults in impoverished communities through literacy education, Friere asserted that hierarchies of power exist between educators and learners. He advocated for democratic relationships, critical examination of existing and accepted assumptions, and collaborative problem-posing dialogue in educational activities.

Praxis, with its emphasis on critical reflection followed by challenge and action, extends the notion of humanizing pedagogies beyond approaches that are friendly, relatable, and rich in demonstrations of immediacy. In health professions education, required disciplinary knowledge, technical skills, and competency-based curricula can reduce, however inadvertently, learning to a series of measurable skills and behaviours (Halman, Baker, & Ng, 2017). In turn, this narrow curricular focus potentially deflects educators' attention away from humanistic pedagogies designed to foster caring, compassionate, and socially responsible health-care providers.

Educational activities geared to questioning and critiquing existing power relations and assumptions, particularly those that could be complicit in perpetuating inequitable and unjust social conditions, might not be supported at system and structural levels (Halman et al., 2017). However, when educators do find ways to integrate the critical reflection inherent in praxis into their teaching, they communicate a willingness to recognize and value learners' perceptions, lived experiences, and questions. Whether learners are novices beginning careers in their chosen professions or expert professionals advancing their knowledge, they need to feel valued and welcomed for who they are. The next strategy suggests a way to value learners for their "fresh views."

A STRATEGY TO TRY

Welcome Fresh Views

In their discussion of critical consciousness as a humanizing pedagogy, Halman et al. (2017) suggest that educators can communicate to learners that they are valued by naming their perspectives as fresh views. When learners are new to an area or topic in health care, they look at practices that others might take for granted with new and fresh perspectives. Inviting learners to express these perceptions (and to critically question the information and practices that they observe) creates a welcoming safe space where knowledge can be exchanged rather than transmitted in a one-way direction.

In clinical practice, novice practitioners might think that they do not have enough knowledge to express their points of view or question existing practices. Knowing that their views have value because they provide new and fresh perspectives can be empowering. Similarly, expert practitioners in new situations can be reluctant to disclose their ideas and critical questions in case disclosure negatively influences their careers. Here again, when instructional activities clearly stipulate that fresh views are welcome and valued, educators create a foundation for establishing and celebrating the kinds of human connections in teaching that can make learners feel "ten feet tall."

Affective Learning

Affect, or how people express emotions and feelings in their communications with others, plays an important role in the education of health professionals. Throughout their careers, they learn and practise in emotionally charged situations. Creating learning environments that embrace the affective nature of health care is a foundational element of humanizing pedagogy.

In his seminal work to classify the domains of learning, educational psychologist Benjamin Bloom (Bloom & Krathwohl, 1956) is credited with identifying three taxonomies of learning: *psychomotor* (physical/kinesthetic), *cognitive* (thinking), and *affective* (emotion/feeling). Health professionals commonly learn psychomotor skills during skills labs and practice sessions; acquire cognitive skills in both classroom and practicum settings; and develop affective skills in collaborative, group, or preceptored experiences. Affective learning is considered a higher level of learning in which understanding the complexities of human connections is essential.

Although a committee of professors and examiners in higher education also contributed significantly to the process of organizing learning into psychomotor, cognitive, and affective domains, the taxonomy is referred to as Bloom's Taxonomy. Revisions of the taxonomy, particularly in relation to affective learning, have continued since the 1950s (Anderson et al., 2000; Anderson et al., 2001; Krathwohl, Bloom, & Masia, 1964).

Educators from a variety of sectors have integrated Bloom's Taxonomy into their teaching. The hierarchical levels identified in each domain provide important guidance in creating learning activities that move from simple to more complex. Most frequently, Bloom's Taxonomy is used to develop outcomes that learners are expected to achieve at the completion of a learning experience.

Five hierarchies have been established in the affective domain: *receiving, responding, valuing, organization*, and *characterization* (Krathwohl et al., 1964). First, at the simplest level, for learners to receive information, they must be aware that a stimulus for learning exists, and they must be willing and receptive to pay attention to this stimulus. Verbs used to describe receiving include *feel, sense, capture, experience, pursue, attend,* and *perceive.* An example of affective learning in the receiving domain is the expectation that students in the health professions attend a practicum placement in which they work under the direction of a preceptor. Learners are present to receive information related to the experience provided.

Second, responding requires learners to pay active attention, demonstrate motivation to learn, and experience feelings of satisfaction with their participation. Here descriptive verbs include *conform, allow, cooperate, contribute, enjoy,* and *satisfy.* When learners in practicum placements go beyond receiving information, they demonstrate responding by working cooperatively with their preceptors and actively contributing to patient/client care.

Third, valuing involves learners integrating information into their own beliefs and values about what they perceive is personally important and valuable. When this level of affective learning occurs, learners express an acceptance of information and show genuine commitment to certain values and beliefs. Descriptive verbs include *believe, seek, justify, respect, search,* and *persuade.* An illustration of valuing is when learners in practicum placements undertake efforts to persuade members of the health-care team to consider a particular treatment approach.

Fourth, organization occurs when learners internalize the personal and professional values that they have begun to conceptualize and include in their thinking. Organization includes establishing priorities based on values. In other words, achieving organization in learning requires that people know what is important to them as well as to their profession. Verbs such as *examine, clarify, systematize, create,* and *integrate* illustrate how the notion of organization reflects an increasingly more complex level of affective learning. When learners in practicum placements converse with others about how they are making connections between what they believe is important and what they are learning from their preceptors and other professionals, they are engaging in this high level of affective learning.

Fifth, characterization occurs when learners act in ways that reflect their internalized values and philosophical views. This high level of affective learning occurs when learners can demonstrate internalization of their own values without compromising expected disciplinary competencies. Verbs used to describe characterization include *internalize, review, conclude, resolve,* and *judge*. An example of characterization in practicum placements is a learner who might not agree with implemented patient/client care. In this example, learners must make judgments about care that they are expected to provide and know when and how to seek the help needed to ensure the safety of those whom they have been assigned to care for.

As Bloom's Taxonomy of affective learning suggests, measuring whether this type of learning is occurring (and at what level) is difficult. Learning experiences in the health professions often include outcomes that indicate an expectation of affective learning. Without human connections to compassionate others, learners might not progress beyond simply attending and responding to requirements of designated activities. When educators focus on the humanizing pedagogies of immediacy, praxis, and affective learning, learners will feel valued for their beliefs and their ways of piecing information together. In turn, this will propel learners to engage in the more complex actions of organizing and characterizing their thinking in new ways.

A STRATEGY TO TRY

Foster Emotional Growth in Learning

When you reflect on the phrase "emotionally charged learning experience," does the memory of a particular learning activity come to mind? The activity could be one that you remember participating in as a learner or an educator. It could be geared to pre-service, in-service, or preceptored learners. The setting could be a face-to-face, clinical, or online classroom. Think about how connecting with other people affected your emotional responses. Which actions did others take to foster your ability to grow and learn in spite of the turmoil that you were experiencing?

Focusing on how human connections can foster emotional growth, apply the five levels of learning described in the affective domain of Bloom's Taxonomy to guide your reflections.

1. Receiving information. When attending the activity, how did educators and others around you let you know that they were present and available to help? What made it easier to find and access information?

2. Responding to information. How did educators recognize and nurture the intrigue that you felt by what you were learning? What actions did they take to support the satisfaction with your progress that you were beginning to feel?

3. Valuing information. Which opportunities were available to share your values, beliefs, and views about the information presented? Whom did you turn to when you felt comfortable enough to share any conflicting views (educator, peer, family member, friend)? Did the available opportunities include options for connecting with people beyond the educational setting? If so, then how was the confidentiality of the health-care setting maintained? How did educators acknowledge that you experienced an emotionally charged response to information? How did they affirm your views? Which strategies did they use to build on those views but still integrate new information?

4. Organizing information. When did you first experience a sense of being able to complete one of the tasks involved in the activity without consciously thinking it through? With whom did you most want to share the feeling of *I can do this*? How did educators create opportunities for you to share your feelings of increasing confidence and emotional growth with peers and fellow professionals? Conversely, when you experienced a sense of feeling stuck and being unable to progress, how did educators help you to connect with more informed others to help you move forward?

5. Characterization of information. Did the activity that you reflected on include a time when a professional commitment did not align with your moral values? Characterization, the highest level of affective learning, might not be present in all learning activities. If characterization was present, then how did you follow through with your values and beliefs while still maintaining patient/client safety?

Conclude your reflections by highlighting educational activities that fostered your emotional growth. Consider ways to include them in your own teaching practice.

In the preceding section, we discussed how environments in which educators and learners are viewed as co-creators of knowledge can celebrate and facilitate human connections in teaching. Next, we extend these ideas by emphasizing the importance of inviting participants in educational experiences to personalize their learning. Clearly, any program that provides education to health professionals must include goals that address content related to required disciplinary knowledge. Traditionally, goals in many programs for both pre-service and in-service learners were geared primarily to the acquisition of systematized skill sets, a relatively finite body of knowledge, and attitudes typically associated with a professional group.

Today, in developed countries around the world, most educational systems have shifted toward more personalized learning in which individuals are also involved in determining the goals that they want to achieve (Ignatovich, 2016). From elementary school to middle school to high school, most students who enter higher education now have some experience setting goals. Guiding learners toward setting personally meaningful goals, giving them the freedom to make choices related to those goals, and helping them to implement relevant problem-solving tools that aid in achieving those goals have emerged internationally as a foundational element in the "democratization and humanization" of all levels of education (Ignatovich, 2016, p. e5).

Personalizing learning focuses on the learner and "refers to instruction that is paced to learning needs, tailored to learning preferences, and tailored to the specific interests of different learners. In an environment that is fully personalized, the [individualized goals] and content as well as the method and pace may all vary" (Bray & McClaskey, n.d.). When the personalization of learning includes individual goal setting, learners can strengthen their individuality, independence, creativity, and competence, and the process can aid them in discovering and developing their humanity (Ignatovich, 2016). Educators in the health professions can no longer focus exclusively on goals stipulated in required curricula. Learners also need opportunities to set goals for themselves and to achieve those goals through means that suit their ways of learning.

My Experience with Personalizing Learning

Reflect on your learning experiences in kindergarten to grade 12, undergraduate, and graduate settings. Were there opportunities for you to personalize your learning? What about your continuing education experiences as a practising health-care professional? What motivated you to go beyond doing just what was required and to extend your learning to include creating personal goals relevant to you? Were there times when you would have liked to personalize your learning but did not? Can you pinpoint what made the difference?

Individual Goal Setting

In educational settings, the expectations of educators and learners are communicated through goal, outcome, and objective statements. According to the Eberly Center (n.d.), goals refer to broad statements about the purpose of a program or course and what *educators* expect learners to achieve over a period of time, outcomes refer to statements about what *graduates* are expected to know and be able to do once they have completed an educational activity or program of study, and objectives refer to specific, measurable statements that describe what *learners* must demonstrate by the end of a course or workshop. In essence, "goals are where you want to go; objectives are how you get there; and outcomes are proof that you have arrived" (Center for Technology, n.d., para. 1).

Differentiating among these different types of statements is important as educators in the health professions consider ways to help learners create individualized goals. At the curricular level, educators in these professions will (and should) always establish the program goals, outcomes, and objectives that will help learners to acquire the skills, knowledge, and attitudes that they need to practise health care safely. However, educators must also remain open to understanding, supporting, and celebrating the goals that learners themselves hope to achieve over time. This process begins when educators establish human connections with their students and intentionally explore what is important and meaningful to them.

When educators actively encourage learners to set individual goals, they nurture the higher-order affective competencies that health professionals need to function effectively in the real world of constantly evolving practice knowledge. In the seminal *Nurse Educator Core Competencies* publication from the World Health Organization (2016, p. 14), "facilitat[ing] professionalization for learners by creating learners'. . . . personal goal setting" is one of the core competencies expected of nurse educators.

Most regulatory bodies and associations in the health professions expect members to establish individualized goals as part of their continuing professional development. Professionals must demonstrate an ability to create and progress toward attaining individual goals throughout their careers. By integrating individual goal setting into experiences for pre-service and in-service learners, educators provide guidance toward succeeding with this professional expectation.

Individual goal setting can help learners with short-term successes in their classes or workshops as well. For example, when pharmacy students were supported with individual goal-setting activities such as creating self-developed study plans and openly discussing their progress toward achieving their goals, they demonstrated significantly improved continuous engagement with learning, improved focus on academic goals, and improved academic performance (Yusuff, 2018). When medical students set individual goals to improve their interviewing skills, they performed better on their Objective Structured Clinical Exams (OSCEs) (Hanley et al., 2014).

Different theories can serve as backdrops for understanding the value of individual goal setting. Notably, in his classic publication *Towards a Theory of Task Motivation and Incentives*, Edwin Locke (1968) theorized that, when people consciously and intentionally set their own goals, they are more motivated to undertake actions that lead to completed tasks. As Locke noted, when people set individual goals, they choose goals that are challenging rather than easy; when those goals are linked to specific tasks, they are more likely to be achieved.

Locke's (1968) thinking lends credence to the notion that educators can help learners to succeed by encouraging them to individualize the goals, outcomes, and objectives identified in their designated curricula. When learners are accountable for their individual goals, that is, when they share them with someone else, they are more likely to succeed (Simon Fraser University, n.d.). With the knowledge that individual goal setting can be highly motivating and lead to successful outcomes, the importance of implementing activities in which learners can practise and become proficient with individual goal setting becomes clear. The strategy below outlines one such activity.

A STRATEGY TO TRY

Why Am I Doing This?

This strategy illustrates individual goal setting by creating links between designated course or workshop goals, objectives, and outcomes and those that are personally meaningful.

Step One

Select a goal, an objective, and an outcome from any course syllabus or workshop that you instruct or participated in as a learner. Note your selections on the left side of a document.

- *Goal:* Prepare graduates to deliver safe, entry-to-practice level care in [a specific clinical area] of [my] profession.
- *Objective:* Achieve a score greater than 80% on the final course/workshop exam.
- *Outcome:* Discuss appropriate clinical data such as history, clinical presentation, and laboratory findings when providing care and communicating with colleagues.

Step Two

Now, on the right side of the document, individualize each of them. Remember that goals are where you want to go, objectives are how you get there, and outcomes are proof that you have arrived.

- Your *goal* will be applicable just to you and where you want to go in your career. Perhaps you have a clinical specialty in which you want to become certified. Highlight how the activities in this course or workshop will help you to move closer to achieving your individual goal.

- Your *objective* will highlight the resources available to you in the course or workshop that you most want to spend time on and master.
- Your *outcome* will illustrate the knowledge, skills, and attitudes that you expect to have developed further by the completion of the learning experience.

Share your completed document with a colleague or employer and integrate it into any professional development/continuing competence records required by your professional association.

Invite learners in your teaching practice to complete the activity as well. Introduce the activity when you explain the goals of the course or workshop. Be sure to check in with learners throughout the course and discuss their progress.

Voice and Choice

When educators provide learners with *voice and choice*, they honour the voices or views of what is important to learners, and they ensure that opportunities for making personally relevant choices are available. The phrase originated in the 1930s when educational systems began to shift toward more democratic education and freedom-based education (Morrison, 2008). These types of education are rooted in a view that people are curious by nature and naturally drawn toward learning, growing, and finding ways to make meaning from their experiences. This curiosity can be diminished when educational practices neglect personal learning.

In contemporary educational settings, the phrase serves as an important reminder for educators to remain vigilant about listening to learners and tuning in to choices that will support their unique learning goals. In pre-service programs offered by institutions of higher education such as universities, learners can choose elective courses of interest to them and might have some flexibility in the sequencing of their courses. Student representatives might be invited to join curriculum planning committees. In pre-service and in-service programs offered by other educational institutions and clinical agencies, learners have fewer choices of courses that they are required to take and when they are required to take them, and they are less likely to be included in planning committees. Many programs in the health professions are time limited and dependent on clinical placement availability.

Despite the limited choices that learners in health care might seem to have at a program level, learner voice and choice can readily be introduced at the instructional level. For example, educators in the health professions are required to deliver content that addresses disciplinary knowledge. All too often a lecture method is used to deliver this content. Similarly, assignment choices are often focused on writing papers or reports. Yet other methods of delivering content and developing assignments are also available. Educators and learners alike can work with multimedia technologies and social media to exchange information and demonstrate understanding of required content in new and exciting ways. Discovering these innovative approaches is most likely to occur when educators express a genuine confidence in learners' capacity to make wise and thoughtful choices.

It is important to emphasize that providing learners with voice and choice also involves thoughtful direction from educators. Learners need to know about options that are (or could be) available to them. They need to know how to access a comprehensive body of required and supplemental resources that will help them to explore their interests and passions. In her work with student teachers, Jackie Gerstein urges educators to "show learners the possibilities . . . and then get out of the way" (n.d., p. 1).

A STRATEGY TO TRY

Assess the Presence of Voice and Choice

Assess whether opportunities for voice and choice were reflected in the assignments for a course or workshop that you developed, taught, or participated in as a learner. Voice refers to what is important to learners, and choice refers to opportunities for learners to make personally relevant choices. Which aspects of the assignments communicated clearly that personalizing learning (choice) was valued and expected in the course or workshop? Can you suggest ways in which the idea of voice and choice could improve these assignments?

CONCLUSION

In this chapter, we invited educators to celebrate the human connections that they can establish and affirm in learning environments. Compassion and humanity are vital in establishing human connections. Humanizing pedagogies, those that emphasize friendliness, immediacy, and affective learning, help educators and learners to work together as co-creators of knowledge. Health professionals must maintain ongoing competence in disciplinary knowledge and best practice guidelines. They must also demonstrate praxis in which they reflect critically and act to transform inequities in these structures. Educational activities in which learners' views and critiques are valued can begin to ameliorate this tension.

Most learners in the health professions now come to programs, courses, and workshops with some experience in personalizing their learning. Educators must intentionally seek ways to strengthen this existing knowledge and help learners to extend their individual goals, objectives, and desired outcomes. Doing so will enhance learning and support professional development. We reminded educators to include voice and choice in the development and instruction of courses and workshops. Voice and choice are particularly important when delivering content and developing assignments in courses and workshops.

In summary, human connections are the heart of successful education in the health professions. Learners, whether they are pre-service or in-service, are continually required to learn new knowledge, new technologies, and new procedures. Educational activities grounded in a genuine commitment to humanizing learning will support learners and help to foster in them a lifelong love of learning.

REFERENCES

Andersen, J. F. (1979). Teacher immediacy as a predictor of teaching effectiveness. *Communication Yearbook, 3,* 543–559.

Anderson, L. W. (Ed.), Krathwohl, D. R. (Ed.), Airasian, P., Cruikshank, K., Mayer, R., Pintrich, P., . . . Wittrock, M. (2000). *A taxonomy for learning, teaching, and assessing: A revision of Bloom's Taxonomy of educational objectives (complete edition).* Boston, MA: Allyn & Bacon.

Anderson, L. W. (Ed.), Krathwohl, D. R. (Ed.), Airasian, P., Cruikshank, K., Mayer, R., Pintrich, P., ... (2001). *A taxonomy for learning, teaching, and assessing: A* revision of Bloom's Taxonomy of educational objectives (abridged edition). Boston, MA: Allyn & Bacon.

Bloom, B. S., & Krathwohl, D. R. (1956). *Taxonomy of educational objectives: The classification of educational goals, by a committee of college and university examiners. Handbook I: Cognitive Domain.* New York, NY: Longmans, Green.

Bray, B., & McClaskey, K. (n.d.). *Personalization vs differentiation vs individualization.* Edmonton, AB: Alberta Education Resources. Retrieved from https://education.alberta.ca/media/3069745/personalizationvsdifferentiationvsindividualization.pdf

Brown, B. (2010). *The gifts of imperfection: Let go of who you think you are supposed to be and embrace who you are.* Center City, MN: Hazelden Publishing.

Center for Technology. (n.d.). *Writing goals, educational objectives and learning outcomes.* Baltimore, MD: Johns Hopkins University.

Dalonges, D., & Fried, J. (2016). Creating immediacy using verbal and nonverbal methods. *Journal of Dental Hygiene, 90*(4), 221–225. Retrieved from http://jdh.adha.org/content/90/4/221.full

Dutton, V. (1976). Humanizing education: A simple definition. *Kappa Delta Pi Record, 12*(3), 79. doi:10.1080/00228958.1976.10516924

Eberly Center. (n.d.). *Goals outcomes objectives.* Pittsburgh, PA: Carnegie Mellon University.

Freire, P. (1970). *Pedagogy of the oppressed.* New York, NY: Continuum.

Gerstein, J. (n.d.). Show learners the possibilities . . . and then get out of the way [Web log post]. Retrieved from https://usergeneratededucation.wordpress.com/2015/07/26/show-learners-the-possibilities-and-then-get-out-of-the-way/

Gorham, J. (1988). The relationship between verbal teacher immediacy behaviours and student learning. *Communication Education, 37*(1), 40–53.

Haar, M. (2018). Increasing sense of community in higher education nursing courses using technology. *Journal of Nutrition Education and Behaviour, 50*(1), 96–99. Retrieved from https://www.jneb.org/article/S1499-4046(17)30234-8/pdf

Halman, M., Baker, L., & Ng, S. (2017). Using critical consciousness to inform health professions education: A literature review. *Perspectives on Medical Education, 6*(1), 12–20. doi:10.1007/s40037-016-0324-y

Hanley, K., Zabar, S., Charap, J., Nicholson, J., Disney, L., Kalet, A., & Gillespie, C. (2014). Self-assessment and goal-setting is associated with an improvement in interviewing skills. *Medical Education Online, 19*, 24407. doi:10.3402/meo.v19.24407

Ignatovitch, A. (2016). Humanization of the learning process in higher educational institutions. *Social Behaviour Research and Practice Open Journal, 1*(2), e5–e7. doi:10.17140/SBRPOJ-1-e00

Kleptsova, E., & Balabanov, A. (2016). Development of humane interpersonal relationships. *International Journal of Environmental and Science Education, 11*(4), 2147–2157. doi:10.12973/ijese.2016.585a

Krathwohl, D. R., Bloom, B. S., & Masia, B. B. (1964). *Taxonomy of educational objectives. Book II: Affective domain.* New York, NY: David McKay.

Lalonde, M., & Hall, L. M. (2016). Preceptor characteristics and the socialization outcomes of new graduate nurses during a preceptorship program. *Nursing Open, 4*(1). doi:10.1002/nop2.58

Lieberman, M. (2014). *Social: Why our brains are wired to connect.* New York, NY: Random House.

Locke, E. A. (1968). Towards a theory of task motivation and incentives. *Organizational Behaviour and Human Performance, 3*(2), 157–189.

Melrose, S., Park, C., & Perry, B. (2013). *Teaching health professionals online: Frameworks and strategies.* Edmonton, AB: Athabasca University Press. Retrieved from http://www.aupress.ca/index.php/books/120234

Merriam-Webster. (n.d.). Compassion. In *Merriam-Webster.com.* Retrieved from https://www.merriam-webster.com/dictionary/compassion

Merriam-Webster. (n.d.). Humanity. In *Merriam-Webster.com.* Retrieved from https://www.merriam-webster.com/dictionary/humanity

Morrison, K. (2008). Democratic classrooms: Promises and challenges of student voice and choice, part one. *Educational Horizons, 87*(1), 50–60. Retrieved from https://eric.ed.gov/?id=EJ815371

Quek, G., & Shorey, S. (2018). Perceptions, experiences, and needs of nursing preceptors and their preceptees: An integrative review. *Journal of Professional Nursing, 34*(5), 417–428. doi:10.1016/j.profnurs.2018.05.003

Salazar, M. (2013). A humanizing pedagogy: Reinventing the principles and practice of education as a journey toward liberation. *Review of Research in Education, 37,* 121–148. Retrieved from http://www.jstor.org/stable/24641959

Simon Fraser University. (n.d.). *Goal setting and accountability.* Student Learning Commons [library resource]. Burnaby, BC: Author. Retrieved from https://www.lib.sfu.ca/about/branches-depts/slc/learning/motivation/goal-setting-accountability

Violanti, M., Kelly, S., Garland, M., & Christen, S. (2018). Instructor clarity, humor, immediacy, and student learning: Replication and extension. *Communication Studies, 69*(3), 251–262. doi:10.1080/10510974.2018.1466718

Vocabulary.com. (n.d.). Humanizing. In *Vocabulary.com Dictionary.* Retrieved from https://www.vocabulary.com/dictionary/humanize

Vocabulary.com. (n.d.). Pedagogy. In *Vocabulary.com Dictionary.* Retrieved from https://www.vocabulary.com/dictionary/pedagogy

Walkem, K. (2014). Instructional immediacy in elearning. *Collegian: The Australian Journal of Nursing Practice, Scholarship and Research, 21*(3), 179–184. doi:10.1016/j.colegn.2013.02.004

World Health Organization. (2016). *Nurse educator competencies.* Geneva, Switzerland: Author. Retrieved from https://www.who.int/hrh/nursing_midwifery/nurse_educator050416.pdf

Yusuff, K. (2018). Does personalized goal setting and study planning improve academic performance and perception of learning experience in a developing setting? *Journal of Taibah University Medical Sciences, 13*(3), 232–237. doi:10.1016/j.jtumed.2018.02.001

2

Valuing Cultural Influences

Through understanding, people will be able to see their similarities before differences.

—Suzy Kassem, 2011, "Truth is Crying".

Our culture is an innate part of who we are as human beings and affects how we relate to other people. Daily, and in all areas of practice, health professionals aid people from a variety of different backgrounds and cultures. Students and patients/clients have different perspectives on and beliefs about how health care should be defined and how it should be provided, and so do we as educators of health professionals. Communicating accurately and respectfully is a vital component of being humane. Inaccurate assumptions, misinterpretations, and limited understandings of cultural influences can result in communication breakdowns. For this reason, we have decided to focus our attention on culture as it affects our ability to be humane and caring. Additionally, learners need to be guided to recognize their own cultural biases and to reflect on how they affect their practice. Culture is in the background of everything that we do as educators and an essential component of both how we teach and what we teach.

Humanizing educators design programs and educational activities so that they prepare professionals who are competent in providing quality care to culturally diverse individuals. Furthermore, educators in pre-service and in-service programs bring their own unique cultural influences to the learning experiences that they develop and facilitate. Few practice and learning environments are composed of homogeneous groups of people from the same culture. Rather, globalization and evolving demographics in most developed countries have led people from different cultural backgrounds to come together in new ways. However, despite their differences, when people from culturally diverse backgrounds come together in settings where health professionals are educated, they share the common goal of wanting to provide the best possible care to patients/clients.

Culture influences the human connections and relationships that educators and learners engage in throughout the process of teaching and learning. An approach that values differences and embraces diversity as a strength lays a foundation for positive humanizing educator-learner relationships (Botelho & Lima, 2020; Day & Beard, 2019; Debs-Ivall, 2018; Zeran, 2016). Hagnauer and Volet's (2014) overview of research on educator-learner relationships in higher education concluded that positive relationships clearly affect learners' successful progress, including factors such as course satisfaction, student retention, learning approaches, and learner achievement. These relationships also have positive effects on educators themselves.

The process of establishing positive relationships between educators and learners, and among participants in learning groups, is affected by multiple factors and contexts (discussed further in Chapter 3). However, culture is a factor that can have a profound effect on how people interact with one another. This is especially apparent in environments in which health professionals learn and work.

In this chapter, we ground our thinking in a belief that any process of valuing cultural influences begins with the humane trait of seeing others as human beings first. In our view, people embrace characteristics that seem to be diverse and hold different ways of looking at the world in high regard. In keeping with the notion that genuinely connecting with people includes an understanding of both their culture and our own, we begin with an explanation of cultural competence by exploring what culture is, what cultural competence involves, the impact of cultural intelligence, the kinds of barriers that can decrease cultural competence, and approaches that can help teachers and learners to overcome barriers in educational settings. We close the chapter with a discussion of aspects of cultural safety and cultural humility relevant to the education of health professionals.

Culture

Culture encompasses the standards, morals, principles, viewpoints, ways of life, and lived experiences shared by a group of people (Sonn & Vermeulen, 2018). Race, ethnicity, age, gender, and sexual orientation all contribute to the diverse cultural identities that individuals and groups affiliate with or have been influenced by (Garneau & Pepin, 2015). Additionally, language, class, religion, spiritual tradition, and immigration status are part of culture (National Association of Social Workers, 2015). Understanding people in relation to their culture(s) provides a view of how they socialize with others and relate to the world around them (Garneau & Pepin, 2015).

People may choose to self-identify with their culture(s), or they may prefer not to do so. It is important to emphasize that not all members of a cultural group necessarily share common characteristics. Stereotyping and failure to identify individual needs can occur when people assume that the values, beliefs, and traditions of a particular group apply to everyone in that group (Williamson & Harrison, 2010).

Culture has been explained as a "system of rules that are the base of what we are and affect how we express ourselves as part of a group and as individuals" (Brownlee & Lee, n.d.). Knowledge of, awareness of, and sensitivity to the kinds of rules that we value ourselves, and those that other people value, comprise an important starting point as educators and learners begin to form relationships.

According to Brownlee and Lee (n.d.), *cultural knowledge* refers to an introductory understanding of some of the cultural history, values, beliefs, and behaviours of a group of people. *Cultural awareness* refers to a somewhat deeper understanding of a group of people and being open to the possibility of changing our attitudes toward that group. *Cultural sensitivity* refers to knowing that differences exist between groups but not assigning values to those differences (e.g., better or worse, right or wrong). When people continue to build and extend their cultural knowledge, awareness, and sensitivity, they can move toward developing cultural competence. We discuss the concept of cultural competence further in the next section. The strategy below invites you to consider ways that you might define your own culture.

The Cultural Group I Most Often Identify with Is. . . .

How would you complete the sentence "the cultural group I most often identify with is. . . ." You might wish to integrate some of the following shared influences that typically affect cultural identification: standards, morals, principles, viewpoints, ways of life, lived experiences, race, ethnicity, age, gender, sexual orientation, language, class, religion, spiritual tradition, and immigration status. Do you self-identify with this cultural group publicly? Why or why not? What impacts do you think your own cultural affiliations have on your teaching practice?

Understanding Cultural Competence

Understanding cultural competence is critical in the complex process of establishing the essential human connections needed for meaningful learning. Explanations of the concept continue to evolve. One seminal multidisciplinary definition by Cross, Bazron, Dennis, and Isaacs (1989, p. 28) states that "cultural competence is a set of congruent behaviours, attitudes and policies that come together in a system, agency or among professionals that enable that system, agency or professionals to work effectively in cross-cultural situations."

In health-care contexts, Betancourt, Green, Carrillo, and Ananeh-Firempong's (2003, p. 293) widely cited definition states that cultural competence is "understanding the importance of social and cultural influences on patients' health beliefs and behaviours; considering how these factors interact at multiple levels of the health-care delivery system; and, finally, devising interventions that take these issues into account to assure quality health-care delivery to diverse patient populations." The need to understand cultural competence becomes increasingly clear when we consider the links between this important concept and truly connecting as teachers with our learners.

Despite a growing acceptance of the importance of cultural competence in health-care delivery and systems of education, individuals continue to receive unequal treatment. In 2002, the seminal report of the Institute of Medicine in the United States—*Unequal Treatment: Confronting Racial and Ethnic*

Disparities in Health Care—identified striking disparities in the health care that non-white minority patients received (Smedley, Stith, & Nelson, 2003). Similar findings have also been reported more recently in Canada, Australia, New Zealand, and Great Britain. In these countries, educational approaches that increase cultural competence in health workforces are viewed as an important step in addressing these pervasive disparities (Jongen, McCalman, & Bainbridge, 2018).

Not unexpectedly, disparities also occur in educational settings (Guerra & Kurtz, 2016; Kruse, Rakha, & Calderone, 2018; Smith, 2018). Successful students in the health professions need culturally competent educators who reflect, value, and celebrate the diverse attributes of the students whom they teach (Abdul-Raheem, 2018; Hunt, 2013; Smith, 2018). Culturally competent educators "adapt teaching and learning techniques in a way that values, empowers, and accommodates . . . student diversity. It begins with an assessment of the learner's needs and includes student interactions, curricula and policy development, in-class and online considerations, culturally competent policies and procedures, and . . . educators committed to lifelong learning" (Smith, 2018, p. 20). In many instances, however, educators can be unsure of how to integrate cultural competence into their teaching approaches, learning environments, and relationships with students (Young & Ramírez, 2017). The following strategy provides a survey that educators can use to open a dialogue with learners about cultural influences important to them.

A STRATEGY TO TRY

"Who Am I" Survey

In *A Nurse Educator's Guide to Cultural Competence*, Smith (2018) encourages educators to open a dialogue with learners about their unique and culturally diverse learning needs with a confidential "Who Am I" survey at the beginning of a learning experience. Smith suggests posing the following questions.

- In addition to being a student, what roles are you now experiencing (spouse, parent, employee), and what's your estimated time commitment to each?
- What are your cultural identities?

- What are your short- and long-term academic and personal goals?
- What is your ideal learning experience?
- What are your learning strengths and challenges?

How might you adapt this survey to assess the diverse needs of learners in your teaching practice? Could this survey be implemented as a sharing circle exercise to promote connections among learners in groups? Do these questions provide opportunities for learners to exchange information about the common culture-related challenges and opportunities that they face? Would facilitating discussions about how learners choose to acknowledge and celebrate their diversity, either individually or in groups, help to develop your own cultural competence?

Cultural Intelligence

Cultural intelligence, also identified as cultural quotient (CQ), refers to people's capacity to relate and work effectively across cultures (Ang & Van Dyne, 2008). People with high cultural intelligence demonstrate a seemingly natural way of relating to others that includes an ability to interpret their unfamiliar and ambiguous gestures, just as members of the other cultural group would, and an ability to differentiate behaviours that are idiosyncratic to someone's individual personality and those that are culturally determined (Earley & Mosakowski, 2004). People with high cultural intelligence are also tuned in to subtle expressions of cultural influence, such as eating rituals, personal space, eye contact, greetings, and tone of voice (Fernandez, 2011). People who enter new cultural groups need cultural intelligence to feel a sense of belonging. Likewise, people who welcome those who are new also need cultural quotient. Across disciplines, educators need cultural intelligence in order to practise cultural competence with learners.

Cultural intelligence is demonstrated through four components: *cognitive, physical, emotional/motivational,* and *metacognitive* (Earley & Mosakowski, 2004). The cognitive component refers to readily available basic information, such as knowledge about beliefs, customs, and taboos common to a culture. People with high cultural intelligence remain aware that this knowledge might not apply to all members of a cultural group. The physical component refers to the actions of people when they communicate with others. This is demonstrated when people mirror the habits and mannerisms that they observe in others from different cultures. Mirroring actions promotes trust and helps others to feel comfortable and accepted. The emotional/motivational component refers to the ways in which people overcome obstacles and demonstrate confidence and self-efficacy in a culture other than their own (Earley & Mosakowski, 2004). The metacognitive component is a more advanced skill that refers to reflective ways of "thinking about one's own thinking." Metacognitive cultural intelligence involves both an awareness of, and critical reflection on, our own assumptions as well as the assumptions that others might have about cultural influences (Chua, Morris, & Mor, 2012). This type of awareness requires people to assess the aspects of their existing cultural knowledge that are most relevant to the situation at hand. Because individuals are able to sift through and organize information from the cognitive, physical, and emotional/motivational components, those with high metacognitive intelligence can determine cultural knowledge likely to be applicable in one situation but not in another. Metacognitive reflection in relation to culture helps people to recognize flaws and gaps in their thinking and leads to continual re-examination and revision of their values and beliefs (Chua et al., 2012).

Scales have been developed to assess cultural quotient. For example, Van Dyne, Ang, and Koh (2008) developed and validated the 20-item CQ scale. This scale (and other resources) are available without cost from the Cultural Intelligence Center (n.d.) in Michigan. You might wish to complete the CQ scale to get in touch with your own metacognitive intelligence.

A STRATEGY TO TRY

CQ Assessment

Assess your own cultural quotient in relation to the following two actions identified in Van Dyne, Ang, and Koh's (2008) 20-item CQ scale.

1. I modify my behaviour to make others more comfortable when I interact with people from different cultural backgrounds.

Barriers to Demonstrating Cultural Competence

Ethnocentrism. One of the barriers to demonstrating cultural competence that exists when people connect and communicate with one another is ethnocentrism. It was first defined by Sumner (1906) as a view that places one's own group at the centre, and everything else is referenced in relation to that view. When people have an ethnocentric view, they are able to interpret behaviours only from their own perspective, and they believe that what is normal for them is normal for everyone else (Rockstuhl & Van Dyne, 2018). Ethnocentric individuals are limited in their ability to be empathetic in relationships with others. Empathy is essential to creating humanizing interactions.

In health care, when practitioners are ethnocentric, or able to provide care only in ways that are normal to them, they alienate patients/clients, misdiagnose problems, provide inadequate treatment, and cannot provide culturally appropriate or competent care. In a Canadian study examining the relationship between ethnocentrism and physical therapists, occupational therapists, and nurses who provide culturally competent care, findings revealed a moderately strong inverse relationship between ethnocentrism and cultural competence (Capel, Dean, & Veenstra, 2008). These researchers called for the inclusion of activities that explore ethnocentrism in courses and workshops in which health professionals learn about (and strengthen) their cultural competence.

Affinity bias. Another barrier that inhibits cultural competence at an interpersonal level is affinity bias. It refers to a preference for associating with others who are like ourselves, whom we can relate to easily, and who make us feel comfortable (Turnbull, 2013). We use the same neural pathways when we think about ourselves and those who are like us, making it easy for us to form relationships with them (Turnbull, 2014).

However, people might not realize that, when they gravitate toward those with similar appearances, backgrounds, and cultural influences, they can inadvertently communicate that this like-minded group of people has greater value. They might not notice that these associations can leave people to whom they do not relate as easily feeling excluded, ignored, and uncared for (Turnbull, 2014). Recognizing affinity bias in ourselves as educators and including opportunities for learners to understand and identify it in themselves, are important in developing cultural competence. If affinity bias causes us to be more cordial toward, caring of, or concerned for others whom we perceive as being like us, then it follows that we might treat others whom we sense are different in a less humanizing way.

Unconscious bias. Bias that we are not conscious of is a further barrier to cultural competence. Studies indicate that our unconscious minds are responsible for at least 80% of our thought processes and decision making (Nalty, 2016). One reason for this is that our brains are processing millions of pieces of information at the same time, and in order for us to make decisions some functions must be automated. The unconscious mind allows people to cope with a fast-paced world and to make decisions while on the move, and unconscious thinking relies on previous experiences so that people can come to conclusions sooner, but it is often missing current context, the unknown, and any newer relevant information (Verghese, 2015).

People can make both conscious and unconscious decisions at the same time. For example, individuals might firmly believe consciously that they do not have any bias toward others because of their social identities. Yet the same individuals might also unconsciously harbour stereotypical and biased attitudes. These attitudes can "unknowingly leak into decision making and behaviours" (Nalty, 2016, p. 45). Although it might not be possible to change the unconscious thinking that leads to biases, as educators we can always make conscious decisions to examine our ethnocentric and affinity biases. Through ongoing efforts to become aware of our attitudes toward other cultures, to take them into account in our interactions, and to work on eliminating them, we can shift our thinking and demonstrate more culturally competent behaviour toward others.

Limited workplace support. Educators and learners also face barriers related to limited institutional support for cultural competence in the workplace. Most learning in the health professions is linked to health service organizations. These organizations might not implement approaches that support culturally competent health-care delivery. In a review of best practices in health service organizations in North America, Australia, and Europe, six approaches to responding to patients/clients from culturally diverse groups were consistently recommended. These approaches are fostering organizational commitment, assessing empirical evidence of inequalities and needs, creating a competent and diverse workforce, ensuring access for all users, maintaining responsiveness in care provision, bolstering patient/client and community participation, and promoting responsiveness (Seeleman, Essink-Bot, Stronks, & Ingleby, 2015).

When health professionals practise and learn in organizations in which recommended approaches have not yet been translated into policies and procedures, they can find it difficult to demonstrate cultural competence. Leaders and co-workers in these organizations might not be fully aware of their personal levels of cultural competence, and they might not view a commitment to improving in this area as a priority. In response, educators can invite learners to explore the construct of cultural competence in their assignments and projects and then encourage them to share what they have discovered with practitioners. In the activity that follows, we invite you to reflect on how bias might affect your own cultural competence.

A STRATEGY TO TRY

Private Reflections

Take a few moments to reflect on how ethnocentric and affinity biases might affect your own cultural competence.

In relation to ethnocentric bias, was there a time when you just assumed that someone else thought the same as you did about a health-care practice? How did you realize that this person did not see the practice as normal?

In relation to affinity bias, have you noticed that it seems to be easier to care for patients/clients or to teach learners who have backgrounds similar to your own? Is it possible that you inadvertently pay more attention to people to whom you feel easily drawn? Might this affinity leave others feeling excluded?

What actions can you take to ameliorate these biases?

In educational systems, barriers to integrating cultural competence exist at system, curricular, and instructional levels. At the educational systems level, higher education and health-care organizations around the world are making efforts to enhance cultural awareness and cultural competence (Hunt, 2013; Peterson, 2019). Examples include initiatives to employ people from different cultures; conduct research in the languages and cultures of diverse people; integrate cultural awareness activities; support student and practitioner organizations that emphasize cultural competence; establish positive relationships between cultural organizations that learners and practitioners have formed and administrative and institutional leaders; and include international studies when possible (Hunt, 2013). In Canada, institutions of higher education such as the First Nations University of Canada in Regina have created programs specifically geared to support Indigenous learners to prosper in their studies and later in their careers. Programs include "Indigenous Healing Practice" and "Indigenous Health Studies" (First Nations University of Canada, n.d.).

At the curricular level, Hunt (2013) suggests direct immersion in another culture by means of an international practicum. Out-of-country field placements provide learners with opportunities to discover universal human characteristics and to appreciate differences in values, beliefs, and attitudes. When the languages that learners speak are different from those of their hosts, non-verbal communication becomes even more essential. Additionally, learners gain new perspectives on the influences that sociopolitical systems exert on health care, and they might view the advantages and disadvantages of their own countries through a different and more informed lens.

At the classroom level, inviting guest speakers from cultures different from those of most of the learners in a group can also promote cultural competence (Hunt, 2013). In both brick-and-mortar and online classroom settings, inviting professionals or patients/clients from different or vulnerable cultures to discuss their values, beliefs, and experiences can evoke lively discussions. Guest speakers provide learners with opportunities to get to know people whom they might not meet otherwise. Sessions can be videotaped for learners to view (or review) independently.

A final and common barrier to integrating cultural competence into health profession programs involves learning resources and course materials with limited diversity content. For example, available textbooks, case studies, simulation scenarios, independent learning modules, slide presentations, podcasts, and videos might not be representative of the cultures and experiences of the individuals and groups expected to use them. The visual images and languages used in learning resources might exclude minority groups or even depict people in these groups in stereotypical ways. The cultural backgrounds of individuals influence their perceptions, and some learners might view information in learning resources as exclusionary, discriminatory, and even racist. The following activity provides an opportunity for educators and learners to review existing learning resources through a lens of cultural competence.

A STRATEGY TO TRY

Resource Review

Gather a selection of learning resources or course materials and invite learners to conduct a resource review. This three-step strategy is suitable for learners in both higher education and continuing education. It can be implemented in face-to-face group settings or in online (synchronous or asynchronous) discussions.

Step one. Introduce the concept of cultural competence and encourage participants to construct a definition personally relevant to them, their own cultures, and their present learning experiences.

Step two. Direct participants to critically review one of the resources (gathered initially) in relation to their definitions of cultural competence and ask them to record instances (or lack) of representation meaningful to them.

Step three. Facilitate a discussion in which the recorded instances are shared among participants. Highlight common themes that emerge. Close the activity with an invitation to continue reflecting critically on existing learning resources and to imagine creating new, inclusive materials that contain equal representations of culturally diverse people.

CULTURAL SAFETY

Cultural safety plays a foundational role in creating the human connections necessary for meaningful education in the health professions. The construct of cultural safety first emerged in the 1980s when it became apparent that the Maori people in New Zealand were not receiving the health care that they needed (Nursing Council of New Zealand, 2002). Since then, the concept has been extended and applied to Indigenous peoples in other countries where service inequalities persist (Yeung, 2016). Cultural safety considers how social and historical contexts, the colonization of Indigenous peoples, and structural and interpersonal power imbalances have shaped people's experiences (Ward, Branch, & Fridkin, 2016).

Self-reflection is a critical component of cultural safety. In this context, self-reflection means continually seeking to understand one's own culture, beliefs, and imprinted stereotypes and considering how they influence attitudes toward others of different cultural backgrounds (Yeung, 2016). The seeking of self-awareness also means reflecting honestly on the power and privilege that one holds in a relationship (Ward, Branch, & Fridkin, 2016).

Culturally safe practices acknowledge inequalities, recognize and respect the cultural identities of others, and safely meet their needs, expectations, and rights. Conversely, culturally unsafe practices "diminish, demean or disempower the cultural identity and well-being of an individual" (Nursing Council of New Zealand, 2002, p. 9). Persons and their families from a particular culture determine whether a practice is culturally safe or not safe for them (Nursing Council of New Zealand, 2002).

When learners participate in educational activities, they should feel confident that the environment in which they are expected to learn is culturally safe. For Indigenous people, this might not always be the case. In higher education, Indigenous people are underrepresented, and the unique challenges that they face as learners might not be recognized (Barney, 2016). Because of underrepresentation, Indigenous learners might not have opportunities to meet and interact with educators who are also Indigenous (Andersen, Bunda, & Walter, 2008).

Indigenous learners might struggle with ill health, family responsibilities, financial issues, cultural isolation, and literacy in ways different from non-Indigenous learners (Andersen et al., 2008; Barney, 2016). In response, some institutions of higher education have supported learner success by creating support services, learning spaces, and orientation programs designed specifically for Indigenous students (Barney, 2016). Unfortunately, many of the institutions that educate pre-service and in-service learners in the health professions are not able to offer these supports.

One Canadian program in nursing offered by the University College of the North (UCN) in Manitoba has integrated these supports (Zeran, 2016). Of the UCN student body, 50% are of Indigenous descent, and like other Indigenous people around the world many experienced feelings of loneliness, alienation, and discrimination when they attended institutions of higher education. Many lacked the educational preparation needed to succeed in a nursing program. In addition to providing academic support, UCN offers support services at Aboriginal Centres located on campus. These centres provide staff and students with opportunities to honour and share cultures, practise cultural beliefs, and promote cross-cultural awareness. "Provisions such as the Elders program, counselling program, role-modelling program, substance-abstinence counselling, family counselling and sharing circles all endeavour to provide a culturally competent and safe learning environment in which students are supported to succeed" (Zeran, 2016, p. 109).

UCN faculty recognized the important role that faculty-student interactions play in recruiting, retaining, and graduating students (Zeran, 2016). In response, they made establishing culturally safe relationships with students a priority. They tried to remain aware of their own cultural influences and to respect the views, values, and beliefs of learners. Indigenous ways of knowing and traditions were threaded throughout the curriculum. All faculty are required to complete an Aboriginal awareness in-service course, and all students are required to complete a "Tradition and Change" course. Both courses introduce participants to traditional Indigenous teachings and cultural practices. Faculty in this program believed that their "caring, sensitive and committed attitude" served as an incentive for their students to be successful (Zeran, 2016, p. 105). In the following strategy, we invite you to reflect on culturally safe spaces in your own teaching practice.

A STRATEGY TO TRY

Culturally Safe Spaces

Think about the experiences of Indigenous learners in the institution or clinical agency where you teach or would like to teach. What might safe spaces look like through their eyes? Which supports are available for this group of learners? Are support services, learning spaces, and orientation programs designed for Indigenous learners (under their direction) available? Are programs available for educators to reflect on their own cultural influences and learn more about Indigenous ways of knowing? How can you find out more about culturally safe spaces in your practice?

CULTURAL HUMILITY

Cultural humility is somewhat different from either cultural competence or cultural safety in that it emphasizes self-humility, self-reflection, and self-critique more than gaining knowledge about other cultures (Tervalon & Murray-García, 1998). In health care, the term "competence" is often conceptualized as mastering a set of skills during a finite period. Tervalon and Murray-García (1998) viewed this conceptualization of cultural competence as illusive and unobtainable. Instead, they suggested that learning about other cultures does not have an end point of understanding and that it is a lifelong process. In their view, cultural humility means considering people's cultures from their individual perspectives and remaining aware and humble enough to "say what [we] do not know when [we] do not know" (p. 119).

Cultural humility has been defined as an "interpersonal stance that is other-oriented rather than self-focused, characterized by respect and lack of superiority toward an individual's cultural background and experience" (Hook, Davis, Owen, Worthington, & Utsey, 2013). In settings where people from different cultures are practising and learning together, cultural humility requires that practitioners and educators view patients/clients/learners as the authorities on their own lived experiences. Cultural humility also requires everyone to remain open to ongoing examination of their own beliefs and biases.

The First Nations Health Authority in British Columbia defined cultural humility as "a process of self-reflection to understand personal and systemic biases and to develop and maintain respectful processes and relationships based on mutual trust. Cultural humility involves humbly acknowledging oneself as a learner when it comes to understanding another's experience" (n.d., p. 7).

The term "cultural humility" has been used in contexts in which individuals have differences in power, ethnicity, race, sexual preference, social status, and interprofessional roles (Foronda, Baptiste, Reinholdt, & Ousman, 2016). Cultural humility has relevance in relationships between health professionals and the patients/clients and learners with whom they engage (First Nations Health Authority, n.d.; Foronda et al. 2016; Chang, Simon, & Dong, 2012; Yeager & Bauer-Wu, 2013). When health professionals demonstrate cultural humility, they can establish humanizing relationships with patients/clients and students that are rich in mutual empowerment, partnership, respect, and support (Chang, Simon, & Dong, 2012).

In learning environments, an understanding of cultural humility can lead to cultural competence (Isaacson, 2014). Of note, cultural humility relates to the compassion inherent in humanity. An individual who displays cultural humility can maintain an interpersonal approach oriented (open) to the other person and what that person views as important (Hook et al., 2013). In such a stance, compassion is a likely outcome.

The process of engaging in honest self-reflection and considering the innate value of each person, foundational to cultural humility, results in a desire to remove inappropriate power imbalances within relationships (Tervalon & Murray-García, 1998). Educators focused on achieving cultural humility view learners as having valuable opinions and knowledge that educators do not possess. Likewise, educators who strive to forge cultural humility in learners help them to recognize that patients/clients are the experts on their own bodies and lives and that they hold knowledge that health professionals do not have. Humanizing approaches to achieving cultural humility focus on learning to collaborate and share expertise.

The following case illustrates a (hypothetical) situation in which a practitioner did not demonstrate cultural humility. Cleaver, Carvajal, and Sheppard (2016) describe the well-intended actions of a physiotherapist who volunteered at a hospital in a low-income country. Drawing on current knowledge of best practices, the physiotherapist interrupted treatment that a local colleague was implementing and suggested an alternative. Cleaver et al. emphasize that the practitioner, who came from a high-income country, did not take context into consideration. The physiotherapist did not ask for any explanation or rationale from the local colleague and did not make any effort to understand the colleague's thinking, which might have been consistent with the realities of the locale.

Like the physiotherapist in the case study, people can overlook the value of cultural humility when they are eager to share their knowledge. Most health professionals are likely to have experienced situations in which practices considered best in one situation were not at all relevant in another situation. The activity below highlights the value of humility in human connections.

A STRATEGY TO TRY

I Meant Well . . .

During discussions with learners, relate a story from your practice in which you meant well, but your actions did not take into consideration the cultural background, knowledge, and experience of a patient/ client, colleague, or learner. Keep the story short and emphasize how a critical self-reflective process led you to a deeper understanding of cultural humility. Individually, or in a group, ask learners to comment on their reactions to the story, and then invite them to share their own experiences.

A primary goal of the strategy is to illustrate information about cultural humility that learners will need to practise in today's multicultural health-care and educational institutions. A secondary but equally important goal is to role-model the process of examining your own beliefs and biases. When educators share brief examples of imperfect practice, and how these practices can begin to be resolved through acknowledgement and change, they invite critical dialogue. Learners are more likely to reflect critically on their own actions and established practice knowledge when they see their teachers actively doing so.

Remaining humble and fully open to others and what is important to them is not easy. Yet professionals, whatever their field of study, are expected to conduct themselves in a manner that is sensitive and respectful toward the cultures, values, and traditions of others. In health care, practitioners, educators, and learners must all engage in continuing efforts to assess and develop their cultural competence, ensure the cultural safety of others, and maintain cultural humility.

CONCLUSION

In this chapter, we explored ways of valuing the cultural influences that shape the complex process of educating health professionals. Educators who model a willingness to understand the influence that culture has on learning can make an important difference. Historically, health professionals have not been responsive to the needs of culturally diverse people. In response, practitioners and educators have made it a priority to understand people in relation to their cultures.

Genuine and reciprocal human connections are most likely to occur in learning environments that foster cultural competence. This competence must include educational approaches that assess and respond to learners in ways that value their individuality and consider aspects of the cultures with which they choose to affiliate. Cultural competence includes remaining knowledgeable about, aware of, and sensitive to cultural influences important to others. It also includes demonstrating cultural intelligence or the ability to work effectively with diverse groups of people. Culturally competent educators also make ongoing efforts to identify and overcome their own biases related to ethnocentricities, affinities, and unconscious thoughts. Such educators actively seek ways to value differences among people and to break down barriers that exist in clinical and educational institutions.

Finally, and perhaps most importantly, culturally competent educators strive to create culturally safe spaces. Learners can experience cultural safety only when educators acknowledge their own cultural beliefs and respectfully meet the needs of learners. Educators, practitioners, and learners must all maintain an attitude of cultural humility in which the practices and beliefs of others are not demeaned or ignored.

REFERENCES

Abdul-Raheem, J. (2018). Cultural humility in nursing education. *Journal of Cultural Diversity, 25*(2), 66–73.

Andersen, C., Bunda, T., & Walter, M. (2008). Indigenous higher education: The role of universities in releasing the potential. *The Australian Journal of Indigenous Education, 37*, 1–8. doi:10.1017/S1326011100016033

Ang, S., & Van Dyne, L. (2008). Conceptualization of cultural intelligence: Definition, distinctiveness, and nomological network. In S. Ang & L. Van Dyne (Eds.), *Handbook of cultural intelligence: Theory, measurement and applications* (p. 3–15). New York, NY: Sharpe.

Betancourt, J., Green, A., Carrillo, J., & Ananeh-Firempong, I. (2003). Defining cultural competence: A practical framework for addressing racial/ethnic disparities in health and health care. *Public Health Reports, 118*(4), 293–302. doi:10.1016/S0033-3549(04)50253-4

Barney, K. (2016). Listening to and learning from the experiences of Aboriginal and Torres Strait Islander students to facilitate success. *Student Success, 7*(1), 1–11. doi:10.5204/ssj.v7i1317

Botelho, M. & Lima., C. (2020). From cultural competence to cultural respect: A critical review of six models. *Journal of Nursing Education, 59*(6), 311-318. doi: 10.3928/01484834-20200520-03

Brownlee, T., & Lee, K. (n.d.). *Section 7: Building culturally competent organizations.* Community Tool Box, Chapter 27. Lawrence, KS: Center for Community and Health Development, University of Kansas. Retrieved from https://ctb.ku.edu/en/table-of-contents/culture/cultural-competence/culturally-competent-organizations/main

Capel, J., Dean, E., & Veenstra, J. (2008). The relationship between cultural competence and ethnocentrism of health care professionals. *Journal of Transcultural Nursing, 19*(8), 121–125. doi:10.1177/1043659607312970

Cleaver, S., Carvajal, J., & Sheppard, P. (2016). Cultural humility: A way of thinking to inform practice globally. *Physiotherapy Canada, 68*(1), 1–2. doi:10.3138/ptc.68.1.GEE

Cross, T., Bazron, B., Dennis, K., & Isaacs, M. (1989). *Towards a culturally competent system of care: A monograph on effective services for minority children who are severely emotionally disturbed.* Washington, DC: Georgetown University Child Development Center, CASSP Technical Assistance Center.

Chang, E., Simon, M., & Dong, X. (2012). Integrating cultural humility into health care professional education and training. *Advances in Health Sciences Education, 17,* 269–278.

Chua, R. Y. J., Morris, M. W., & Mor, S. (2012). Collaborating across cultures: Cultural metacognition and affect-based trust in creative collaboration. *Organizational Behaviour and Human Decision Processes, 118*(2), 116–131. Retrieved from https://ink.library.smu.edu.sg/lkcsb_research/3964

Cultural Intelligence Center. (n.d.). *Cultural Intelligence Centre* [website]. https://culturalq.com/products-services/assessments/

Day, L., & Beard, K. (2019). Meaningful inclusion of diverse voices: The case for culturally responsive teaching in nursing education. *Journal of Professional Nursing, 35*(4), 277–281. doi:10.1016/j.profnurs.2019.01.002

Debs-Ivall, S. (2018). Do you value difference and embrace diversity as a strength? *The Canadian Nurse, 114*(3), 44.

Earley, P. C., & Mosakowski, E. (2004). Cultural intelligence. *Harvard Business Review, 82*(10), 139–146. Retrieved from https://pdfs.semanticscholar.org/7242/bb07d3f9568f1579d5e0d87f189a673c5c65.pdf

Fernandez, G. A. (2011). Do you know your cultural IQ? *Franchising World,* 16–18.

First Nations Health Authority. (n.d.). *#itstartswithme: Creating a climate for change.* Victoria, BC: Author. Retrieved from http://www.fnha.ca/Documents/FNHA-Creating-a-Climate-For-Change-Cultural-Humility-Resource-Booklet.pdf

First Nations University of Canada. (n.d.). *Welcome to First Nations University of Canada.* Retrieved from http://fnuniv.ca/

Foronda, C., Baptiste, D., Reinholdt, M., & Ousman, K. (2016). Cultural humility: A concept analysis. *Journal of Transcultural Nursing, 27*(3), 210–217. doi:10.1177/1043659615592677

Garneau, A. B., & Pepin, J. (2015). Cultural competence: A constructivist definition. *Journal of Transcultural Nursing, 26*(1), 9–15. doi:10.1177/1043659614541294

Guerra, O., & Kurtz, D. (2016). Building collaboration: A scoping review of cultural competency and safety education and training for healthcare students and professionals in Canada. *Teaching and Learning in Medicine, 29*(2), 129–142. doi:10.1080/10401334.2016.1234960

Hagenauer, G., & Volet, S. (2014) Teacher–student relationship at university: An important yet under-researched field, *Oxford Review of Education,* 40(3), 370-388, doi: 10.1080/03054985.2014.921613

Hook, J., Davis, D., Owen, J., Worthington, E., & Utsey, S. (2013). Cultural humility: Measuring openness to culturally diverse clients. *Journal of Counseling Psychology, 60*(3), 353–366. doi:10.1037/a0032595

Hunt, E. (2013). Cultural safety in university teaching and learning. *Procedia Social and Behavioural Sciences, 106,* 767–776. doi:10.1016/j.sbspro.2013.12.088

Isaacson, M. (2014). Clarifying concepts: Cultural humility or competency. *Journal of Transcultural Nursing, 30*(3), 251–258. doi:10.1016/j.profnurs.2013.09.011

Jongen, C., McCalman, J., & Bainbridge, R. (2018). Health workforce cultural competency interventions: A systemic scoping review. *BMC Health Services Research, 18,* Article 232. doi:10.1186/s12913-018-3001-5

Kassem, S. (2011). *Rise up and salute the sun: The writings of Suzy Kassem.* Boston: Awakened Press.

Kruse, S., Rakha, S., & Calderone, S. (2018). Developing cultural competency in higher education: An agenda for practice. *Teaching in Higher Education, 23*(6), 733–750. doi:10.1080/13562517.2017.1414790

Nalty, K. (2016). Strategies for confronting unconscious bias. *The Colorado Lawyer,* 45(4), 45–54. Retrieved from https://kathleennaltyconsulting.com/wp-content/uploads/2016/05/Strategies-for-Confronting-Unconscious-Bias-The-Colorado-Lawyer-May-2016.pdf

National Association of Social Workers. (2015). *Standards for cultural competence in social work practice*. Washington, DC: Author.

Nursing Council of New Zealand. (2002). *Guidelines for cultural safety, the treaty of Waitangi, and Maori health in nursing and midwifery education and practice*. Wellington, New Zealand: Nursing Council of New Zealand.

Peterson, C. (2019). Fostering cultural humility among nursing students in a global health setting. *Nurse Educator, 44*(2), Article 111. doi:10.1097/NNE.0000000000000575

Rockstuhl, T., & Van Dyne, L. (2018). A bi-factor theory of the four-factor model of cultural intelligence: Meta-analysis and theoretical extensions. *Organizational Behaviour and Human Decision Processes, 148*, 124–144. doi:10.1016/j.obhdp.2018.07.005

Seeleman, C., Essink-Bot, M., Stronks, K., & Ingleby, D. (2015). How should health service organizations respond to diversity? A content analysis of six approaches. *BMC Health Services, 15*, Article 510. doi:10.1186/s12913-015-1159-7

Smedley, B., Stith, A., & Nelson, A. (2003). *Unequal treatment: Confronting racial and ethnic disparities in health care*. Washington, DC: National Academies Press.

Smith, L. (2018). A nurse educator's guide to cultural competence. *Nursing Made Incredibly Easy, 16*(2), 19–23. doi:10.1097/01.NME.0000529955.66161.1e

Sonn, I., & Vermeulen, N. (2018). Occupational therapy students' experiences and perceptions of culture during fieldwork. *South African Journal of Occupational Therapy, 48*(1), 34–39. doi:10.17159/2310-3833/2017/vol48n1a7

Sumner, W. (1906). *Folkways: A study of the sociological importance of usages, manners, customs, mores, and morals*. Boston, MA: Ginn.

Tervalon, M., & Murray-García, J. (1998). Cultural humility versus cultural competence: A critical distinction in defining physician training outcomes in multicultural education. *Journal of Health Care for the Poor and Underserved, 9*(2), 117–125. doi:10.1353/hpu.2010.0233

Turnbull, H. (2013). *Inclusion, exclusion, illusion and collusion: Helen Turnbull at TEDxDelrayBeach* [Video file]. Retrieved from https://www.youtube.com/watch?v=zdV8OpXhl2g

Turnbull, H. (2014, May 20). The affinity bias conundrum: The illusion of inclusion part III. *Profiles in Diversity Journal*. Retrieved from http://www.diversityjournal.com/13763-affinity-bias-conundrum-illusion-inclusion-part-iii/

Van Dyne, L., Ang, S., & Koh, C. (2008). Development and validation of the CQS: The cultural intelligence scale. In S. Ang & L. Van Dyne (Eds.), *Handbook of cultural intelligence: Theory, measurement and applications* (p. 16–38). New York, NY: Sharpe.

Verghese, T. (2015). *Developing your cultural intelligence* [Video file]. Retrieved from https://www.youtube.com/watch?v=UAcHUIRwQUo&feature=youtu.be

Ward, C., Branch, C., & Fridkin, A. (2016). What is Indigenous cultural safety and why should I care about it? *Visions BC's Mental Health and Addictions Journal, 11*(4), 29–32. Retrieved from http://www.heretohelp.bc.ca/sites/default/files/visions-indigenous-people-vol11.pdf

Williamson, M., & Harrison, L. (2010). Providing culturally appropriate care: A literature review. *International Journal of Nursing Studies, 47*(6), 761–769. doi:10.1016/j.ijnurstu.2009.12.012

Yeager, K., & Bauer-Wu, S. (2013). Cultural humility: Essential foundation for clinical researchers. *Applied Nursing Research, 26*(4), 251–256. Retrieved from https://www.ncbi.nlm.nih.gov/pmc/articles/PMC3834043/

Yeung, S. (2016). Conceptualizing cultural safety: Definitions and applications of safety in health care for Indigenous mothers in Canada. *Journal for Social Thought, 1*(1), 1–13. Retrieved from https://pdfs.semanticscholar.org/90b0/a619eb b52a2663c731d4ca22cbb1c48a8cc1.pdf

Young, A., & Ramírez, M. (2017). I would teach it but I don't know how: Faculty perceptions of cultural competence in the health sciences, a case analysis. *Humboldt Journal of Social Relations, 39*, 90–103. Retrieved from https://digitalcommons.humboldt.edu/cgi/viewcontent.cgi?article=1024&context=hjsr

Zeran, V. (2016). Cultural competency and safety in nursing education: A case study. *The Northern Review, 43*, 105–115. Retrieved from https://thenorthernreview.ca/index.php/nr/article/view/591/626

3

Enhancing Relationships Among Educators and Learners

No significant learning can occur without a significant relationship.

—James Comer, 1995

Culturally competent relationships make the difference (Trottier, 2016). More specifically, humanizing relationships enhance many aspects of life, including formal and informal teaching-learning situations. Learning experiences in the health professions generally involve interacting with others. The interactions can occur in face-to-face as well as online settings. Relationships can take place formally in programs offered by university and technical institutions or in orientation and staff development programs offered by clinical agencies. Or interpersonal relationships can develop informally when people need to know more about a concept and do so by exchanging information with peers and informed others.

Whether learners are novice pre-service students in higher education or expert in-service clinicians extending their expertise through further education, in most instances they will be required to communicate with others. Similarly, whether learners are engaged in formal programs of study or working independently to achieve and update competencies, there will be times when they interact with others. All too often these interactions do not develop into humanizing relationships. Rather, they remain task-oriented interactions geared to simply delivering and receiving information.

In our view, superficial interactions among people can develop into genuine relationships only when human connections are made. In other words, relationships deepen and become reciprocal when they are humanized. It is a challenge to define precisely and clearly what is meant by the term "humanizing" (when it is applied to relationships among learners, educators, and fellow learners) even though it is used freely in the educational literature. Humanism is considered everything from a philosophy or an attitude to a political stance or an intellectual position (Létourneau, Cara, & Goudreau, 2017). Edwards, McArthur, and Russell-Owens (2016) edge toward a definition of humanization in learning experiences by describing such environments as judgment-free zones in which learners are encouraged to freely share, reflect, and question.

Theories such as the I-Thou Relationship (Buber), Person-Centred Approach (Rogers), and Ingredients of Caring (Mayeroff) are founded on humanism. Themes such as mutual growth in relationships because of reciprocity, caring behaviour, and attitudes that influence this mutual growth, the existence of growth potential in all individuals, and journeying together through learning (growth) experiences are common to all of these theories (Létourneau et al., 2017). Values such as respect, dignity, compassion, and honesty seem to be foundational to humanism-based theories and the formation and maintenance of humanizing relationships.

Such relationships in the variety of learning experiences that health professionals participate in are grounded in these themes and values. Furthermore, relationships that can be considered humanizing establish beneficial exchanges among educators and learners. They require authenticity of intentionality and commitment among educators to do what they can to create affirming environments in which learners' voices are encouraged and acknowledged. As Bartolomé (1994, p. 173) explained, humanization in education is an approach that "values the students' background knowledge, culture, and life experiences, and creates learning contexts where power is shared by students and teachers."

Educators who nurture humanizing relationships between themselves and their students actively pursue a path toward "mutual humanization" (Freire, 1970). A mutual and humanizing relationship welcomes shared ownership among educators and students and views learners as co-investigators instead of receivers of information (Yosso, 2005). Humanizing educators encourage engaging in emotional dialogue, sharing (even clashing) of views, and storytelling (Reyes, 2016). Educators demonstrate humanizing relationships when they view learners as co-creators of knowledge instead of empty vessels that need to be filled.

In this chapter, we focus on humanizing approaches that can help educators to create and enhance these kinds of humanizing relationships. We begin by introducing the community of inquiry (CoI) model (see Figure 3.1), elements of which illustrate a useful frame of reference that educators can use to cultivate connections with students and among participants in learning groups. We then integrate this model into a discussion of three significant relationships in learning environments: those between educators and learners, those between learners and learners, and those that learners cultivate outside the classroom. We conclude the chapter with a discussion of innovative approaches that can help educators to foster these relationships and make them matter.

Community of Inquiry

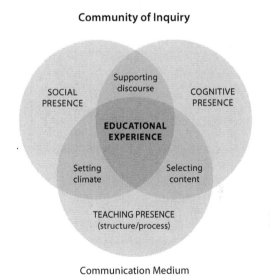

Figure 3.1 Elements of an educational experience. Source: Garrison, Anderson, & Archer, 2000.

The CoI model provides a simple and concise visualization of three key elements present in most educational experiences. These experiences usually include facilitators or teachers who provide guidance, other learners who provide a sense of community, and opportunities for learners to reflect on and make sense of information. The CoI model named these three elements teaching presence, social presence, and cognitive presence (Anderson, Rourke, Garrison, & Archer, 2001; Garrison, Anderson, & Archer, 2000; Garrison, Anderson, & Archer, n.d.).

Although the model was initially designed as a tool for computer-mediated communication in online learning environments in higher-education settings, educators in other practice areas can also apply the elements to their teaching. Creating a community of inquiry by addressing teaching presence, social presence, and cognitive presence and by considering how they overlap are hallmarks of education in all learning environments (Garrison et al., n.d.). When educators establish a robust community of inquiry, they can create, nurture, and maintain relationships with and among learners.

TEACHING PRESENCE

The first element of the CoI model is teaching presence, defined as "the design, facilitation, and direction of cognitive and social processes for the purpose of realizing personally meaningful and educationally worthwhile learning outcomes" (Anderson et al., 2001, p. 1). Inherently, when students experience the presence of the teacher who provides the structure of cognitive direction and the process of human interaction, a climate of openness and a sense of community in the class are facilitated. Educators demonstrate teaching presence by providing guidance, building understanding, and motivating learners (Anderson et at., 2001). Teaching presence is viewed by students as foundational to helpful student-teacher relationships.

At the curricular level, teaching presence is reflected in the way that a course or workshop is designed or organized and begins even before educators meet learners. Learners can feel well supported when they see clear links among course goals, curricular materials, expected outcomes, learning activities, and assessment measures (Anderson et al., 2001). Although many educators in the health professions are not directly involved in designing the courses and workshops that they facilitate, they can and should pay special attention to ensuring that learners understand what they are expected to achieve. Educators who convey teaching presence help participants to navigate learning experiences and make sense of course or workshop content.

At the instructional level, educators can establish teaching presence effectively when they facilitate "collaborative dialogues with other participants (peers and teachers) through discussions that personalize, challenge, and expand on the topics covered in class" (Pearson Higher Education Services, n.d., p. 3). Educators can stimulate this critically important dialogue by posing questions, focusing discussions, moderating learner participation, and finding areas of consensus (Pearson Higher Education Services, n.d.).

Teaching presence is also demonstrated when educators provide specific direction. Learners sense that educators are genuinely present when they share their own ideas, suggest resources, make abstract concepts more concrete, connect concepts, provide frequent feedback, and correct learners' misconceptions (Pearson Higher Education Services, n.d.).

Educators can communicate that they are present and involved by sharing content in a conversational rather than an academic style (Pearson Higher Education Services, n.d.). The words that educators use can communicate a willingness to share ownership of the learning process with learners. Humanistic relationships rich in shared ownership and emotional dialogue are grounded in mutual understanding.

In some instances, educators and learners might not fully understand one another. This might be partly the result of different uses of language and colloquial expressions. When educators use only academic terms or their own ways of speaking to share knowledge, they can inadvertently exclude contributions from learners. In their exploration of humanizing relationships between educators and learners, Edwards et al. (2016) revealed that, when educators included words and colloquialisms that learners were familiar with and used themselves, they created important bonds that helped to establish mutual understanding and trust.

The following strategy suggests an approach that educators can use to gain a deeper understanding of the unique word choices important to learners. When educators use vocabulary that learners can understand easily, they are better equipped to provide the structured directions and to facilitate the processes needed to demonstrate teaching presence.

A STRATEGY TO TRY

Language Choice Matters

Educators who seek to create humanizing relationships with learners need to listen to the language used by learners. Astute educators look for common colloquialisms or words that learners substitute for academic terms with which educators are most comfortable.

Educators who learn and use (appropriately) the language of the health professionals whom they are guiding can help to create bonds that establish mutual trust. In turn, this trust can help relationships to move from superficial interactions to more genuine humanizing relationships.

In their research exploring humanizing relationships among educators and learners different from them, Edwards et al. (2016, p. 430) noticed that learners (young girls) were "swapping out common expressions for some of [the educators'] scholarly language of academese." When the educators intentionally used some of the girls' terms, a "sisterhood" developed, and the relationships between educators and learners deepened.

As a strategy, consider recording one of your classes and then review the recording, looking carefully for specific words that learners use. In your next class, strengthen your teaching presence by integrating these words into your teaching and observing the learners' reactions.

COGNITIVE PRESENCE

The second element in the CoI model is cognitive presence, "the extent to which the participants in any particular configuration of a community of inquiry are able to construct meaning through sustained communication" (Anderson et al., 2001, p. 1). There is overlap among the three elements. For example, cognitive presence (i.e., critical, practical inquiry) can be formed by effective teaching presence and social presence (Garrison, Anderson, & Archer, 2001).

Cognitive presence is grounded in the ever-evolving relationship between personal meaning and shared dialogue. When people feel curious or puzzled and have questions, they often begin to find answers through personal inquiry, reflection, and integration of resources available to them. This practical process of inquiry can lead to thinking more critically when people include collaboration with others. When they explore issues and exchange ideas together, they can integrate information differently, find alternative ways to construct meaning, and then apply their new knowledge (Garrison et al., 2001). Cognitive presence is associated with higher-order knowledge acquisition and application: "Cognitive presence is a process of inquiry that includes thinking, listening and expressing thoughts in the process of critical discourse. It is a collaborative process of thinking and learning in deep and meaningful ways" (Garrison, 2017, p. 3).

The cognitive presence of the teacher is a core concept in creating a community of inquiry (Garrison et al., 2001). It is through their cognitive presence that educators select content to be emphasized and how they support the kind of discourse that can bring that content to life. Educators who have effective relationships with learners can challenge them to think critically, provide additional examples from practice, and improve the quality of their assignments. Communication, a mainstay of cognitive presence, both cultivates educator-learner relationships and helps them to mature in a way that enhances learning. The following activity illustrates how educators and learners can share the responsibility of maintaining a strong cognitive presence in their learning experiences.

A STRATEGY TO TRY

Learner-Led Case Study Discussions

Case study discussions are used frequently in health education programs. Often the cases, a series of questions, and reference materials are provided to educators, who typically lead the discussions. Consider shifting the leadership of cases to a learner or learner pair. Provide them with the case and materials ahead of time. Ensure that all members of the group have an opportunity to lead a case discussion at some point in the course/workshop.

As a participant in rather than a leader of the discussion, focus on integrating new information when necessary and making connections among the ideas generated by the group. Highlight perspectives introduced by group members that were not included in the materials provided.

Close the activity by summarizing (with the student leaders) how the original information provided in the case materials was extended as a result of the group discussions. Highlight how the discussions

> moved beyond simply answering questions about what to do toward
> a deeper understanding of what the patient/client depicted in the case
> study might have been experiencing.

SOCIAL PRESENCE

The third element in the CoI model is social presence, "the ability of learners to project their personal characteristics into the community of inquiry, thereby presenting themselves as 'real people'" (Rourke, Anderson, Garrison, & Archer, 2001, p. 51). When members of learning groups risk sharing their views and who they are as people, the dynamics of the group can develop and progress.

Categories of social presence include emotional expression, open communication, and group cohesion (Garrison et al., 2000). The category of emotional expression has been explored further, and an addition to the CoI model could be emotional presence, defined as "the outward expression of emotion, affect, and feeling by individuals and among individuals in a community of inquiry, as they relate to and interact with the learning technology, course content, students, and the instructor" (Cleveland-Innes & Campbell, 2012, p. 283). Emotions influence learning, and educators should recognize, examine, and seek ways of understanding the critical role that emotions play in learning (Cleveland-Innes & Campbell, 2012).

When learning experiences are rich in all of the categories of social presence, participants define discussion topics, encourage collaboration, and initiate discussions (Garrison et al., 2000). Educators can facilitate social presence by setting climate and supporting discourse (Rourke et al., 2001).

In the fast-paced world of health-care delivery and education, questions can be raised about the importance of cultivating social presence in learning environments. Pre-service and in-service learners can view the idea of getting to know others in their learning group and collaborating with them on projects as less important than achieving the competencies required by their discipline. With this view in mind, we highlight that the CoI model emphasizes that

> the primary importance of [social presence] is as a support for cognitive
> presence, indirectly facilitating the process of critical thinking carried on
> by the community of learners. . . . [When] learners find interaction in the

group enjoyable and personally fulfilling . . . they remain . . . in the program, [which] directly contributes to the success of the educational experience. (Garrison et al., 2000, p. 89)

From a social constructivist point of view, learning is shaped by context, and people learn from each other (Vygotsky, 1962). Learners are more likely to engage with their education (Kuh, 2009) and persist with their studies when they feel connected to, and involved with, other members of the learning community (Tinto, 1993). Interacting, collaborating, and communicating with peers can help individuals in a learning group to make sense of information presented and to find alternative ways of constructing personal meaning. Research has consistently demonstrated that, when learners experienced high perceptions of social presence in their learning environments (particularly in online settings), they felt more satisfied with their learning experiences (Alsadoon, 2018; Cobb, 2011; Horzum, 2015; Gunawardena & Zittle, 1997); they also felt more satisfied with their teachers (Richardson & Swan, 2003). Therefore, social presence is important in learner engagement, persistence, satisfaction, and meaning creation.

Social presence is likely the most fundamental element of the creation of learners' relationships with other learners and with educators. Models of teaching and learning that feature interaction and engagement with others help to create social presence. It can be experienced when learners and educators project themselves socially and affectively into the learning milieu. Any activities that help learners and educators to get to know each other, to sense a connection to the group, and to feel that they are not alone can contribute to social presence (Plante & Asselin, 2014). When educators create opportunities for participants in learning experiences to share in-depth self-introductions, to offer meaningful support to peers' goals, and to collaborate on projects, they foster social presence. The strategy below can be used to help identify values that members of a group have in common.

A STRATEGY TO TRY

A Professional I Admire Is . . .

Invite participants in a roundtable discussion in a 10–15-member learning group to finish the sentence "a professional I admire is. . . ." As participants share information about the health professionals whom they admire, draw out characteristics that they describe. For example, you might say "you mentioned that [the professional] took time to listen carefully to her patient/client. It sounds as though empathy is important to you. Are there others in the group who also feel this way?"

Keep the discussion moving and ensure that all participants have equal time to speak. The strategy can be used in face-to-face or online settings and with pre-service and in-service learners.

RELATIONSHIPS IN LEARNING ENVIRONMENTS

The CoI model described in the previous section can be helpful as a theoretical foundation to guide the development of humanistic relationships in learning environments. Teaching presence, cognitive presence, and social presence can all enhance connections among educators and learners, and we ground the discussion that follows on these presences. Although there are many different associations that can emerge when people participate in learning experiences, we focus on the kinds of meaningful relationships that learners can establish with educators (educator-learner), with fellow learners (learner-learner), and with knowledge that they glean independently from a variety of sources (relationships outside the classroom). Some also consider student–course content a relationship dyad, whereas others consider student-self a relationship. However, since the focus of this book is on the essential *human* connections that make such a critical difference in the education of health professionals, we discuss the first three pairs.

Educator-Learner

Educator-learner relationships are vital to successful teaching and learning (Hershkovzt & Forkosh-Baruch, 2017). Success in teaching and learning includes both achievement of learning outcomes and development of less tangible and less measurable emotional, social, and psychological outcomes. Research on student achievement (learning outcomes) by Hattie (2012, p. 5) concluded that "what teachers do matters," and for some students relationships with teachers can "tip the scale away from academic failure and move students toward scholastic success." In Hanson's (2018) study, the influence of the student-teacher relationship emerged as the catalyst for fostering student resilience and academic achievement. As Trottier (2016) concludes, when teachers connect with their students, it helps them to build social, emotional, and academic skills.

In some circumstances, a relationship in which the educator acts as a mentor or role model leads to a positive future for a learner both personally and professionally (Theron & Engelbrecht, 2012). As Hansen (2018, p. 30) writes, "many students, despite abysmal circumstances, thrive emotionally and socially due to the resilience-building power of teachers."

What can educators do to cultivate resilience in learners? It begins with creating connections with learners (most possible in a humanizing learning environment). Once connections are established, educators are more able to cultivate internal factors such as humour, optimism, and flexibility in learners. These traits make learners less vulnerable to frustration, hopelessness, and feelings of defeat that can undermine their scholastic achievement and professional success.

A STRATEGY TO TRY

Building Resilience: Create a Risk-Approved Classroom

Resilience is like a muscle to be developed. Learners who never make mistakes or never fail are not likely to develop strong resilience. To help learners build resilience, openly discuss the value of failure. Reassure learners that creativity (and its associated risk) are requisite elements of assignments, and when they do take a chance with class work or in discussion take note and appreciate their attempts. What you praise shows what you value. Include marks for ingenuity (even if the product by some measures is a disaster).

Collaborations. In many ways, humanizing educator-learner relationships are collaborations, which call for equal contributions from all parties in a relationship. To contribute requires participation, and participatory learning is aligned with humanizing pedagogy (Gleason, 2017). Successful collaborations between educators and learners were found to lead to open dialogue, positive relationships, and the establishment of a learning community; moreover, such successful collaborations can be catalysts for change in learners, educators, and even the institutions in which they learn and work (Wang & Kao, 2013).

Beaton (2017) described how an educator-learner collaboration model resulted in educators coming to better understand individual learner's interests, creative abilities, and varied learning needs. Beaton emphasized the need for active participation by both parties for a successful collaboration to emerge and be sustained. The optimal outcome for such a collaboration is a community of shared learning. Beaton concluded that, just as learners thrive in a safe, engaging, and collaborative learning environment, so too do educators.

Collaborations, within a humanizing milieu, can fuel the development, achievement, and energy of educators and learners alike. Strategies that value learners' background knowledge, culture, life experiences, and approaches that create learning contexts in which power is shared equally are important in developing effective educator-learner relationships. Collaborative learning environments depend on the authenticity of intentionality and commitment by the educator. The strategy below suggests a way in which educators can promote collaboration in learning groups by inviting participants to share what they are interested in and feel passionately about.

A STRATEGY TO TRY

Tell Me About You

Most successful collaborations happen when collaborators are well acquainted with one another. This strategy is a variation of grade school days Show and Tell. Ask learners to share a personal artifact with the group that reveals their interests or passions. The artifacts can be as varied as the participants are but can include a selection of music, a photograph, or a piece of clothing. The essential element of the strategy is that learners also share what the artifact means to them and why they chose it to represent their interests and passions. For this exercise to be the foundation of a collaboration, educators also participate by sharing one of their most significant artifacts.

Learner-Learner

Relationships among learners are also important for positive academic or professional development experiences. Constructive relationships among classroom or workshop colleagues are the foundation for the establishment of a sense of community in the group. When learners feel a sense of community, they believe that they belong, and the belief that every member of the classroom is valued is shared by all participants (Lloyd, Kolodziej, & Brashears, 2016). Haney, Thomas, and Vaughn (2011, p. 56–57) also discovered that building a classroom community "fosters belonging rather than isolation" among students. When learners interact in respectful ways, meaning that their interactions are guided by empathy, fairness, self-control, and tolerance, it is possible to build a healthy learning milieu in which all participants feel safe to engage in active learning.

Where the elements of teaching, cognitive, and social presences in the CoI model intersect is the educational experience of the learner. When the experience includes this sense of community, the learner-to-learner relationships are both facilitated and enhanced. Educators can use purposeful strategies to foster a sense of belonging in learners even if they are learning in seeming isolation, such as working through an independent online module. The first step might be to focus on creating social presence or the sense that individuals are "real" (Garrison et al., 2001).

Creating a sense of community requires a foundation of trust and respect among participants, and it takes time to develop. Educators who value forging strong learner-learner relationships devote time and effort to helping class members know that they are learning in a safe space and that there are others in the class who respect and value their contributions. All learners need to be recognized and valued for their unique abilities, interests, and skills. Some factors that can inhibit learners from creating helpful relationships with their peers include insecurity about their value and abilities. When people feel insecure, experience failure, or have low self-esteem, they can resist trying new things, taking risks, or participating in activities fully. To create a healthy learning community in which valuable relationships are nurtured, full participation by all is fundamental. The next strategy can help to strengthen learner-learner relationships by fostering a sense of belonging among learners.

Fostering Belonging Rather than Isolation

Any strategy that helps learners to find their voices, builds their self-esteem, and invites them to share their talents and skills with the class or learning group can remind learners that they are important members of a vital community. One way to achieve this is to have your group work together (or in small break-out groups) to develop a "bill of rights and rules for the class." This list of rights and rules will likely include statements about the value of each person and reinforce the appreciation of diversity and the worth of each voice. Throughout the learning experience, the educator (and participants) can refer to this document to support initiatives or help to correct instances when the bill is violated.

Outside the Classroom

As the world becomes the classroom for learners, people have opportunities to interact with teachers other than those leading/guiding the formal classes, workshops, or orientation programs in which they are registered. These informal educators can range from mentors who work with learners in professional settings to experts with whom learners interact virtually through an online community of practice. Although these informal teachers have no jurisdiction over formative or summative feedback or specified learning outcomes and activities, they are becoming increasingly important elements in learning relationships and collaborations.

These "connectivity opportunities," which exist in part because learners have access to teachers/mentors anywhere in the world through digital means, can aid learners in the development of critical thinking and inquiry. As Garrison (2016, p. 1) writes, we need to "rethink conventional education in light of technological developments," and the unprecedented access that learners now have to multiple "teachers" can lead to even deeper and more meaningful learning. Ubiquitous communication technology allows learners and educators (both formal and informal) to connect and develop relationships that support dialogue and reflection that are foundational to learning. The strategy that follows illustrates how relationships in learning environments can occur outside the classroom.

Mentor-mentee relationships. One type of educator-learner relationship that can occur outside a formal learning situation is mentoring. It is defined as the process of helping and advising a younger, less experienced person (Cambridge Dictionary, n.d). Humanizing mentor-mentee relationships can change the professional and personal well-being of both participants. The mentoring relationship takes on the quality of a shared learning journey in which both people can benefit. Mentees can benefit as mentors help them to recognize and believe in their abilities, hone their skills, help them to network and connect with others who can benefit their careers, and act as a confidant and an anchor during difficult times.

Reverse mentoring is somewhat different from traditional mentoring. According to Murphy (2012), reverse mentoring involves a younger and junior person who shares expertise with an older and senior person. As Murphy notes, reverse mentoring was first introduced in 1999 when senior managers at General Electric were paired with younger employees instructed to teach them about the internet. Since then, organizations have implemented reverse mentoring as a way of tapping into the technical knowledge of younger workers, fostering cross-generational learning, and developing leaders among the younger "anchor" generation.

In both traditional and reverse mentoring relationships, mentors often gain knowledge and skills from their interactions with mentees. Aspects of mentoring relationships can lead mentees to reflect on taken-for-granted practices, collect feedback on their teaching approaches, be inspired, and remain relevant in their professions.

There are several types of mentors according to Fawal (2018). One is a "master of the craft," a person who has accumulated wisdom over years of experience and is positioned to guide a more inexperienced person. Another type of mentor is considered a "champion" of the mentee. That type of mentor advocates for a more junior person and aids his or her career by making introductions to others who might help to move his or her learning and work forward. A third type of mentor, the "co-pilot," takes on a collaborator role with the mentee in which both parties support one another and hold each other accountable. The anchor type often does not have specific disciplinary knowledge but acts as a confidant and helps to lift in spirits in challenging times. In the following strategy, we suggest how educators can use Twitter as a mentoring tool.

A STRATEGY TO TRY

Twitter Mentor

To start, educators can invite learners to find a Twitter mentor relevant to a class or workshop topic. For example, if the topic is nursing leadership, then learners might seek out the Twitter feed of a respected national or local nursing manager and follow that feed to determine the priorities, approaches, and problems accompanying that person. Students can interact with the person whom they are following through questions and comments. The strategy could include a formal written analysis of what the learner discovered about the course topic from the Twitter mentor experience.

Effective relationships of all types (educator-learner, learner-learner, or with "teachers" outside the classroom) are deepened by actions and strategies that emphasize the human connection in the dyad. Simply put, by humanizing relationships, we make them matter (or at least make them matter more). Educators and learners who seek to develop and sustain relationships that advance their learning, and provide satisfying interactions, can take deliberate steps to find success in this pursuit. Furthermore, humanizing pedagogy supports the idea that creating opportunities for educators and learners to engage in meaningful dialogue and work collaboratively and share reciprocity within an environment of caring behaviours and attitudes, can enhance learning for all parties.

The following section outlines a series of approaches that educators can implement to make the relationships in their learning environments matter. These approaches can be implemented in a variety of educational settings (online, academic classrooms, clinical practice areas) and are relevant to both pre-service and in-service learners. Some of these approaches have been created for and tested by practising educators in the health professions, others are from the literature, and still others are founded on learning theory but have yet to be tested in the real world. The common denominator of these approaches is that they help to create in participants (educators and learners of all types) an increased awareness of mutual connection and interdependence. In one way or another, all of these approaches are focused on humanizing relationships among educators and learners. We encourage educators to regard being and voice, to challenge and disrupt curricula, to make theory real, to share a little bit of you, to reach out with gratitude, to think and communicate in a humanizing way, to demonstrate care and empathy, and most of all to remain fully present with learners.

Regard Being and Voice

To create and sustain humanizing relationships, there must be an unquestioned regard for the being and voice of each participant. Educators must shed (or at least become aware of and set aside) any preconceived views and biases of gender, race, age, background, and other cultural influences. Doing so sets the stage for teachers to engage in relationships with learners that focus on achievement rather than on any preconceived inadequacies or stereotypes (Edwards et al., 2016). In other words, respect for each learner, fuelled by an underlying belief in, and appreciation for, the present contribution and future potential of that person is the foundation for a humanizing relationship. Encouraging each learner to find and use her or his voice, and then truly listening to each person (listening not just with the ears but also with the heart), comprises the basis of positive humanizing teaching-learning relationships.

Storytelling—more precisely, sharing stories one to one or in a learning group—can help people to find their voices and share their truths and realities. As San Pedro, Carlos, and Mburu conclude, we "co-construct these realities in the space between the telling and hearing of stories," with the outcome being "humanizing and more fertile spaces" where our commonalities help to sustain meaningful relationships (2017, p. 667). The strategy using a photostory described below is one technique that can produce poignant outcomes.

A STRATEGY TO TRY

Photostory

To facilitate the sharing of personally meaningful stories, create an instructional strategy using digital photos. Ask learners to compile a slide show of digital images that reflects one memorable or formative time in their personal or professional lives. Learners can use their own images or locate appropriate photos from an open source photo site such as Flickr. The photostory can be accessorized with music or voice-over narration. Music selections are also available for free download from sites such as Jamando. Educators can create a gallery of the photostories so that learners can view one another's compositions. As with all sharing strategies, it is important for educators to create and share their own photostories with their classes to help create connections and enact the idea that the learning journey is shared.

Challenge and Disrupt Curricula

In traditional teaching-learning situations, a carefully crafted curriculum—including predetermined learning resources, learning activities, and assessment approaches—can shut down authentic learning and destroy individualization. Learners might feel obligated to spout what the teacher wants to hear to achieve "success" and pass the required academic course or professional development activity. When educators provide a platform for learners to achieve individual learning outcomes important to their personal and professional lives through learning strategies that fit their learning styles, there is an openness in the learning space that encourages personalization. When this openness includes encouraging learners to display achievement of their learning outcomes in a way meaningful to them, the potential for genuine sharing and relationship building emerges.

Educators who value a humanized learning environment include teaching approaches that help them to learn about the talents, existing knowledge, and special skills of each student. There are many ways to achieve this, and it is often an ongoing effort throughout a course or workshop. For example, learning about the uniqueness of each student begins during the introduction activity in an educational experience. Skilled educators ask questions that help learners to disclose their abilities and talents without feeling as if they are boasting. Questions such as "can you tell us one surprising thing about you?" or "what was the moment in your life that you felt most proud?" often provide opportunities for learners to comfortably share one of their talents with the group. Once this information is disclosed, a skilled educator shows respect for the information and finds ways to value it during the course. It can be as simple as remembering that a specific learner had a talent in art and inviting that person to capture a complex course or workshop concept in a drawing for the class. This approach enhances individual self-confidence, shows respect for the learner, and fuels openness to doing things differently within the course and curriculum.

Respecting the individual is the first step in developing humanizing relationships, and educational design and content that can be moulded to fit the individual (in terms of both process and product) are essential for demonstrating respect. The more educators and course designers can match the curriculum, course, instructional and assessment strategies, and feedback to the individual learner, the greater the potential for all involved to have humanized learning encounters. In the strategy below, we discuss how contracted learning can begin to challenge and disrupt curriculum.

Contracted Learning

To personalize learning, set up a learning contract with each participant in a learning experience. Learners are provided with the overarching outcomes that have been designated, but the approach to achieving them (as well as a specific learning focus) is individualized. At the outset of the course or workshop, learners create a number of learning outcomes that they believe will allow them to meet the designated outcomes but are geared to their own learning priorities. These personalized outcomes are shared with the educator, and a negotiated contract signed by both results. There are many variations of the contracted learning strategy, and the contract can include independent learning (i.e., learners may oversee locating appropriate resources and designing assessment activities to demonstrate achievement of their learning outcomes, or they may simply set up personalized learning outcomes that educators will guide them to achieve).

Make Theory Real

Educators in professional fields want to ensure that learners not only understand theory and the frameworks that guide practice but also become skilled at applying them in their own disciplines and work lives. Moving from theory and the abstract to human and the real in heath care is essential. As Wrenn and Wrenn wrote, "there is nothing more practical than a good theory" (2009, p. 258). Professional programs for health professionals must prepare participants to function as practitioners in their specializations. This process usually involves both class and field or placement experiences.

To make theory to practice educational experiences effective, learners need to be active. Active learning means that participants do more than simply listen to an educator; they also undertake activities that focus on skill development and achievement of higher-order cognitive learning domain outcomes such as evaluation, critique, and analysis.

Educators need to create and use strategies that help learners to become active and create connections between theory and practical learning experiences. Of course, these learning experiences (to show respect for learners) need to be of interest and importance to them. Inviting learners to move outside the class or workshop to learn in their own daily environments is one approach. In this way, learners construct meaning through their own experiences and discoveries and are challenged to look for ways to apply theory that they mighty have studied in class to their real worlds.

The world outside the classroom is immense. It can include the workplace, social media, and personal and family interactions. One activity that involves the workplace application of theory is to ask learners to memo a question related to course content on their phones and then to ask their colleagues the question during a coffee break at work. In a course on leadership in the health professions, learners were asked to memo the question "can you describe examples of transformational leadership that we experience daily on our clinical unit?" When learners ask this question of their colleagues over coffee, they must be able to explain transformational leadership theory to them. That way their colleagues can answer the question. But they must also evaluate the answers of others. To provide this explanation of the theory and to adequately assess the answers provided aid learning and help to make theory real for learners.

With ready access to social media, the world becomes a potential classroom. One specific activity used in a health policy course involves inviting learners to find and follow (on social media) someone from a national organization who has responsibility for developing or enacting health policy. Learners follow this person over a period of time and then analyze the themes and findings related to policy theory demonstrated by this individual. Again, theory becomes real. As outlined in the strategy that follows, another strategy is to invite a guest speaker to help make theory real for learners.

A STRATEGY TO TRY

Make Theory Real

Invite to the class or workshop a guest speaker who is an expert practitioner on a course topic. The guest can be in person or via electronic means. Invite learners to ask questions of the guest and engage in conversation and large group discussion. Focus the questions and discussions on the translation of theory into practice by asking about examples of what works (and what does not work) in the field.

Share a Little Bit of You

Appropriate self-disclosure can help learners and educators to identify commonalities that foster the formation of bonds and relationships. Self-disclosure is rooted in humanist psychology and is defined as "the act of making yourself manifest, showing yourself so that others can perceive you" (Jourard, 2017, p. 17). More specifically, educators' self-disclosure includes "statements in the classroom about the self that may or may not be related to the subject content but reveal information about the teacher that students are unlikely to learn from other sources" (Sorensen, 1989, p. 259).

When learners enter classrooms or workshops, they know very little about their educators or others in their learning groups. Setting up opportunities for learners (and educators) to be open about personal topics such as hobbies, personal flaws, or past failures or successes can help relationships to emerge. It takes someone in a relationship to go first, for self-disclosure usually takes place within the context of previous self-disclosure. As Henry and Thorsen (2018) note, in "established relationships, inferences made following another person's self-disclosure are interpreted within the relationship's history." An educator who shares stories and experiences demonstrates to learners that it is acceptable to disclose such information. This is one way to create honest sharing as a norm in a learning experience.

In mentoring relationships, this can be an especially effective strategy for teaching by personal example while also forging bonds. When an educator shares a story about a weakness or personal failure, it can open the door for the learner to feel comfortable sharing a similar personal experience. This sharing can evolve into a sense that we are all human and have all had similar experiences. This helps to create a truly collaborative space where participants can reflect, share, and question openly. Henry and Thorsen (2018), in a study focusing on the "relationality" of educator-learner relationships and the role that educator identity disclosure has in enhancing relational practice, found that self-disclosure increased learners' motivation and helped to shape relationships in positive ways. The next strategy notes how effective self-disclosure can be a valuable way of sharing a little bit of you.

Reach Out with Gratitude

Letters of gratitude comprise one strategy that could actively cultivate a mentoring relationship. This approach was used successfully in an online course in which learners were to create a relationship with a mentor to help them continue to develop personally and professionally. The learners were encouraged to write letters of gratitude to people in their lives (present or past) who had helped to shape their attitudes, values, and beliefs in positive ways. In their letters, they shared details of how those people had influenced them. Once the letters were shared, earlier relationships were often rekindled, and enduring mentoring relationships resulted.

Letters of Gratitude

Invite learners to recall people in their lives who helped to shape them into the persons whom they have become. It could be a former teacher, coach, religious leader, relative, or family friend. Tell learners to write letters to these people describing specific incidents that they remember and what those incidents meant to them. The letter could be a written note, an email, or a social media message and should be rich with gratitude. Learners should be encouraged to deliver their "letters" if possible. Host a discussion in the class or workshop about some of the incidents and mentors that learners recalled and share responses that they received to their letters.

Think and Communicate in a Humanizing Way

Educators who create humanizing learning environments think and communicate in a humanizing way. All of their actions and interactions are founded on values that support, encourage, challenge, and respect the dignity and potential of every learner. Humanizing educators are not afraid to show compassion for a learner who struggles because they are committed to the success of each participant in the group (even if "success" means dropping out of the learning experience if that is the right thing for that learner). Humanizing thinking includes showing confidence in learners' abilities (even when learners doubt themselves) and challenging learners to achieve greater learning outcomes than they initially thought possible. Such educators provide learners with opportunities to "fix" things if they are struggling with a concept or an assignment, and they find ways to help learners stay focused on achieving their individualized learning goals.

Being a humanizing educator is vital to relationships with learners. Through modelling, educators can teach important lessons related to being a humanizing professional. Health professionals care for human beings, who are not objects to be manipulated but people who need care and compassion. Humanizing educators can instill this message in part through their own actions and interactions with learners.

One specific strategy that can help learners who are struggling is finding (and teaching) ways to improve on rather than criticize deficiencies. With written assignments in settings of higher education, feedback that includes examples of the "right" way to structure a sentence rather than writing "unclear" in the margin, or providing an example of correct format for a citation rather than saying "marks off for citation errors," enhances learning and humanizes the learning environment. Also related to feedback is the intentional use of positive language. Educators who use negative words when providing feedback or interacting with learners demotivate and dehumanize them. Conversely, educators who choose motivating words that include at least some phrases that acknowledge success and effort create a positive climate in which learners can feel successful. Positive language is an important aspect of any successful educator-learner relationship.

A STRATEGY TO TRY

Humanizing Communication Analysis

Communicating in a humanizing way starts with considering the question "how do I like to be treated?" The golden rule. In this activity, the educator develops several realistic patient/client scenarios that end with the question "what would you say?" Learners work in small groups and review the scenarios and address the question in discussions with group members. After each person in the group answers the question, the group engages in an analysis of the responses to assess how humanizing (or not) each was.

Demonstrate Caring and Empathy

All participants in learning situations are people. Successful people achieve all five levels of Maslow's hierarchy of needs (McLeod 2018), including safety and security, the need to belong, and esteem needs of achievement and accomplishment. An educator who creates a humanizing learning environment includes strategies that help learners to achieve these basic human needs. When an educator shows caring and empathy through actions and words, learners feel safe and are more open to trying learning activities even if they fear that they might fail in them. They know that the educator will acknowledge their attempts and find ways to help them improve rather than simply criticize their work.

Furthermore, humanizing educators know that learners need to feel that they belong and are contributing members of the group. In response, these educators deliberately set up activities in which learners work in teams to achieve a goal. They look for opportunities to comment on a learner's contribution to the group, and they make that person feel that she or he is an important part of the learning community. Finally, helping learners to fulfill the need for achievement and success is a priority for caring educators. All learners face myriad challenges in their lives that can distract them from educational success. Humanizing educators take time to learn about these distractions and challenges and provide learners with support, understanding, and strategies to cope and succeed even in adverse situations.

In an extreme example, one student was facing death from a debilitating disease that rendered it impossible for her to type her final assignment in her final course in a university program of studies. The educator came to know of this reality and created an alternative assignment for the learner (an audio-recorded "paper") that helped her to succeed and meet the course requirements. After the student died, the educator contacted the university registrar and included the student's partner in the graduation ceremony, at which the student's degree was presented posthumously. This is an example of a humanizing educator who demonstrated compassion and empathy. The strategy that follows highlights how educators can use videos to bring demonstrations of caring and empathy into learning experiences.

A STRATEGY TO TRY

Videos of Caring and Empathy

A strategy for teaching caring and empathy involves sharing and analyzing videos (YouTube, movies, movie trailers, TV, etc.) that depict moments when these values are enacted. Learners can be asked to find, share, and analyze these moments independently, or the educator can share a selected movie/video with the group and engage in a discussion related to these themes. Many of them can be located online. Some examples are

- *It's the Great Pumpkin, Charlie Brown*
- *Humans of New York*
- *The Elephant Man*
- *The Grapes of Wrath*
- *Pay It Forward*

Remain Fully Present

Finally, as the above approaches grounded in the CoI model illustrated, remain fully present with learners. Guide and structure learning experiences that genuinely foster human interaction (teaching presence). Ensure that opportunities exist for individuals to create personal meaning through shared dialogue (cognitive presence). Model open communication and establish a welcoming climate in which people can risk being themselves and learn with and from one another (social presence).

When educators are fully present and establish a humanizing learning environment, learners gain the knowledge, skills, and attitudes that contribute to their success in many aspects of life. Educators have the power to create and sustain a humanizing learning milieu. To do so requires consistent commitment and deliberate action. Importantly, educators must find ways to communicate to learners that they are committed to them and their learning. This is often part of an initial interaction with learners as a class or workshop begins. Whether in a lecture hall, an orientation session with new employees, or an introductory video or statement in an online class, educators can communicate through sincere verbal (and non-verbal) expressions that they want to be fully present, that they are real and human, and that they care about learners. However, educators cannot simply tell learners once at the start of a course or workshop that they are committed to supporting them. Rather, they must remain fully present during interactions throughout the learning experience. We expand on this notion in Chapter 4, in which we discuss ways that educators can infuse humanity into different aspects of a curriculum.

Part of remaining fully present involves recognizing that relationships in learning environments, like all relationships, are fragile. Poorly considered or careless comments and actions conveying that educators are not present and committed to learners can have a strikingly negative effect. Effective teaching depends on an educator's ability to achieve social and emotional connections with learners (Gkonou & Mercer, 2017). As we have emphasized throughout this book, humanizing connections lead to positive relationships that can have a significant impact on learning motivation and achievement. However, these connections can be damaged or severed by inconsiderate words and actions from an educator. Even though it might be unintended, a momentary lapse in educator engagement can irreparably damage relationships with learners.

CONCLUSION

In this chapter, we explored approaches that enhance relationships between educators and learners. The CoI model provides a theoretical foundation that educators in different settings can implement to foster relationships between educators and learners and among participants in learning groups. The CoI model consists of three elements: teaching presence, cognitive presence, and social presence. Teaching presence requires educators to direct learners toward relevant outcomes. Cognitive presence requires educators to support learners in constructing personal meaning through individual reflection and group discourse. And social presence requires educators to ensure that all members of learning groups (educators and learners) project their personalities and who they are as people into the learning community. Together, these three types of presence can help to create and sustain the essential human connections that health professional learners value in their educational endeavours.

Relationships in learning environments include those between educators and learners, among members of learning groups, and between students and "teachers" outside the classroom. Educator-learner relationships support learners' achievement and success, particularly when the relationships are collaborative. Learner-learner relationships (in which members of a learning group feel a sense of belonging to the community and a connection with other participants) help people to persist with and succeed in their studies. Relationships in which learners engage with informal teachers and mentors outside the classroom, and from anywhere in the world through digital means, offer unexpected and exciting new ways for people to create meaning.

Finally, we emphasized practical approaches that educators can implement in everyday practice to make relationships matter. When educators regard being and voice, challenge and disrupt curricula, make theory real, share a bit of themselves, reach out with gratitude, think and communicate in a humanizing way, demonstrate caring and humanity, and remain fully present with learners, they humanize their relationships. Enhancing relationships between educators and learners can be as simple as remaining "real" throughout learning experiences and authentically attending to teaching, cognitive, and social presence.

REFERENCES

Alsadoon, E. (2018). The impact of social presence on learners' satisfaction in mobile learning. *The Turkish Journal of Educational Technology, 17*(1), 226–233. Retrieved from https://files.eric.ed.gov/fulltext/EJ1165749.pdf

Anderson, T., Rourke, L., Garrison, D. R., & Archer, W. (2001). Assessing teaching presence in a computer conference environment. *Journal of Asynchronous Learning Networks, 5*(2), 1–17.

Bartolomé, L. (1994). Beyond the methods fetish: Toward a humanizing pedagogy. *Harvard Educational Review, 64*(2), 173–195. doi:10.17763/ haer.64.2.58q5m5744t325730

Beaton, A. M. (2017). Designing a community of shared learning. *Educational Leadership, 74*(8), 78–82. Retrieved from http://0-search.ebscohost.com.aupac.lib. athabascau.ca/login.aspx?direct=true&db=rch&AN=122879082&site=eds-live

Cambridge. Mentoring. (n.d.). In *Cambridge dictionary*. Retrieved from https:// dictionary.cambridge.org/dictionary/english/mentoring

Cleveland-Innes, M., & Campbell, P. (2012). Emotional presence, learning, and the online learning environment. *The International Review of Research in Open and Distributed Learning, 13*(4), 269–292. doi:10.19173/irrodl.v13i4.123

Cobb, S. C. (2011). Social presence, satisfaction, and perceived learning of RN-to-BSN students in web-based nursing courses. *Nursing Education Perspectives, 32*(2), 115–119. doi:10.5480/1536-5026- 32.2.11

Comer, J. (1995). Lecture given at Education Service Center, Region IV. Houston, TX.

Edwards, E., McArthur, S. A., & Russell-Owens, L. (2016). Relationships, being-ness, and voice: Exploring multiple dimensions of humanizing work with black girls. *Equity & Excellence in Education, 49*(4), 428–439.

Fawal, J. (2018). The 5 types of mentors you need in your life. Retrieved from https:// ideas.ted.com/the-5-types-of-mentors-you-need-in-your-life/

Freire, P. (1970). *Pedagogy of the oppressed*. New York, NY: Continuum.

Garrison, D. R. (2016). *E-learning in the 21st century: A community of inquiry framework for research and practice*. London, UK: Routledge.

Garrison, D. R., (2017, September 5). Cognitive presence and critical thinking [Editorial]. Retrieved from http://www.thecommunityofinquiry.org/editorial5

Garrison, D. R., Anderson, T., & Archer, W. (n.d.). Critical thinking and computer conferencing: A model and tool for assessing cognitive presence. Retrieved from https://core.ac.uk/download/pdf/58774863.pdf

Garrison, D. R., Anderson, T., & Archer, W. (2000). Critical inquiry in a text-based environment: Computer conferencing in higher education. *The Internet and Higher Education, 2*(2–3), 87–105. Retrieved from http://cde.athabascau.ca/coi_site/documents/Garrison_Anderson_Archer_Critical_Inquiry_model.pdf

Garrison, D.R., Anderson, T., & Archer, W. (2001). Critical thinking, cognitive presence, and computer conferencing in distance education. *American Journal of Distance Education, 15*(1), 7-23. doi:10.1080/08923640109527o7 *(16) (PDF) Critical Thinking, Cognitive Presence, and Computer Conferencing in Distance Education*. Available from: https://www.researchgate.net/publication/245816834_Critical_Thinking_Cognitive_Presence_and_Computer_Conferencing_in_Distance_Education

Gleason, B. W. (2017). The world of teenage Twitter: New literacies, identity work, and humanizing pedagogy. *Dissertation Abstracts International: Section A. Humanities and Social Sciences, 77*(12-A) (E), 2017. Retrieved from http://o-gateway.proquest.com.aupac.lib.athabascau.ca/openurl?url_ver=Z39.88-2004&rft_val_fmt=info:ofi/fmt:kev:mtx:dissertation&res_dat=xri:pqm&rft_dat=xri:pqdiss:10144339

Gkonou, C., & Mercer, S. (2017). Understanding emotional and social intelligence among English language teachers. *ELT Research Papers, 17.03.* London, UK: British Council Retrieved from https://www.researchgate.net/profile/Sarah_Mercer2/publication/312475321_Understanding_emotional_and_social_intelligence_among_English_language_teachers/links/58a076baaca272046aad5c54/Understanding-emotional-and-social-intelligence-among-English-language-teachers.pdf

Gunawardena, C., & Zittle, F. (1997). Social presence as a predictor of satisfaction within a computer-mediated conferencing environment. *American Journal of Distance Education, 11*(3), 8–26. doi:10.1080/08923649709526970

Haney, K. G., Thomas, J., & Vaughn, C. (2011). Identity border crossings within school communities, precursors to restorative conferencing: A symbolic interactionist study. *School Community Journal, 21*(2), 55–80. Retrieved from http://www.schoolcommunitynetwork.org/SCJ.aspx

Hansen, T. (2018). All because of my teacher: A practical approach to developing positive student-teacher relationships. *Leadership, 47*(4), 30–34.

Hattie, J. (2012). *Visible learning for teachers: Maximizing impact on learning.* London, UK: Routledge.

Henry, A., & Thorsen, C. (2018). Teachers' self-disclosures and influences on students' motivation: A relational perspective. *International Journal of Bilingual Education and Bilingualism*. https://doi.org/10.1080/13670050.2018.1441261

Hershkovzt, A., & Forkosh-Baruch, A. (2017). Teacher-student relationship and Facebook-mediated communication: Student perceptions. *Comunicar, 25*(53), 91–100. doi:10.3916/C53-2017-09

Horzum, M. (2015). Interaction, structure, social presence, and satisfaction in online learning. *Eurasia Journal of Mathematics, Science and Technology Education, 11*(3), 505–512. doi:10.12973/eurasia.2014.1324a

Jourard, S. M. (2017). *Self-disclosure: The experimental investigation of the transparent self.* New York: Wiley.

Kuh, G. D. (2009). What student affairs professionals need to know about student engagement. *Journal of College Student Development, 50*, 683–706.

Létourneau, D., Cara, C., & Goudreau, J. (2017). Humanizing nursing care: An analysis of caring theories through the lens of humanism. *International Journal for Human Caring, 21*(1), 32–40. Retrieved from http://0-search.ebscohost.com. aupac.lib.athabascau.ca/login.aspx?direct=true&db=rzh&AN=125469869&site= eds-live

Lloyd, M. H., Kolodziej, N. J., & Brashears, K. M. (2016). Classroom discourse: An essential component in building a classroom community. *School Community Journal, 26*(2), 291–304.

McLeod, S. (2018). Maslow's hierarchy of needs. Retrieved from https://www. simplypsychology.org/maslow.html

Murphy, W. (2012). Reverse mentoring at work: fostering cross-generational learning and developing millennial leaders. *Human Resource Management, 51*(4), 549–574. doi:10.1002/hrm.214

Pearson Higher Education Services. (n.d.). *Teaching Presence* [White paper]. Retrieved from https://www.pearsoned.com/wp-content/uploads/INSTR6230_ TeachingPresence_WP_f.pdf

Plante, K., & Asselin, M. (2014). Best practices for creating social presence and caring behaviours online. *Nursing Education Perspectives, 35*(4), 219–223. doi:10.5480/13-1094.1

Reyes, III, R. (2016). In a world of disposable students: The humanizing elements of border pedagogy in teacher education. *High School Journal, 99*(4), 337–350. Retrieved from http://0-search.ebscohost.com.aupac.lib.athabascau.ca/login.aspx ?direct=true&db=a9h&AN=114852045&site=eds-live

Richardson, J. C., & Swan, K. (2003). Examining social presence in online courses in relation to students' perceived learning and satisfaction. *Journal of Asynchronous Learning Networks, 7*(1), 68–88.

Rourke, L., Anderson, T., Garrison, D. R., & Archer, W. (2001). Assessing social presence in asynchronous, text-based computer conferencing. *Journal of Distance Education, 14*(3), 51–70.

San Pedro, T., Carlos, E., & Mburu, J. (2017). Critical listening and storying: Fostering respect for difference and action within and beyond a Native American literature classroom. *Urban Education, 52*(5), 667-693. https://doi. org/10.1177%2F0042085915623346

Sorenson, G. (1989). The relationship among teachers' self-disclosive statements, students' perceptions, and affective learning. *Communication Education, 38,* 259–276. doi:10.1080/03634528909378762

Theron, L. C., & Engelbrecht, P. (2012). *Caring teachers: Teacher-youth transactions to promote resilience.* In M. Ungar (Ed.), *The social ecology of resilience: A handbook of theory and practice* (p. 265–280). Springer Science + Business Media. https://doi.org/10.1007/978-1-4614-0586-3_21

Tinto, V. (1993). *Leaving college: Rethinking the causes and cures of student attrition* (2nd ed.). Chicago, IL: University of Chicago Press.

Trottier, P. A. (2016). *Relationships make the difference: Connect with your students and help them build social, emotional and academic skills.* Markham, ON: Pembroke Publishers.

Vygotsky, L. S. (1962). *Thought and language.* Cambridge, MA: MIT Press. (Original work published 1934).

Wang, L., & Kao, Y. (2013). Teacher-student collaboration on designing instructional multimedia materials. *Pacific-Asian Education Journal, 25*(1), 63–75. Retrieved from http://0-search.ebscohost.com.aupac.lib.athabascau.ca/login.aspx?direct=tr ue&db=ehh&AN=111632975&site=eds-live

Wrenn, J., & Wrenn, B. (2009). Enhancing learning by integrating theory and practice. *International Journal of Teaching and Learning in Higher Education, 21*(2), 258–265.

Yosso, T. (2005). Whose culture has capital? A critical race theory discussion of community cultural wealth. *Race, Ethnicity and Education, 81,* 69–91. doi:10.1080/1361332052000341006

4

Infusing Curricula with Humanity

The curriculum is so much necessary raw material, but warmth is the vital element for the growing plant and for the soul.

—Carl Jung, 2014, p. 17

Curricula refer to different educational and instructional practices. A curriculum, the singular form of curricula, is a formal plan of study that provides the philosophical underpinnings, goals, and guidelines for delivery and evaluation methods that a specific educational program will implement (Keating, 2015).

In his seminal article "What Is Curriculum?" Egan (1978, 2003) explained that the word derives from the Latin *currere*, which carried directly over into English, and means "running a race [or a] course," with a secondary meaning of running around a racetrack (1978, p. 10). The metaphor of running a race suggests that curricula, like racetracks, have predetermined structures clearly in place. Curricular structures include explicit plans for learners to interact with instructional content and processes and for evaluating the attainment of educational goals.

In higher-education settings, the academic content of a curriculum is a foundational element of most learning experiences. Additionally, an informal curriculum—the activities that students, faculty, administrators, staff, and consumers experience outside the academic curriculum—is part of the overarching curricula in higher education. Examples of an informal curriculum include interpersonal relationships, athletic/recreational activities, study groups, organizational activities, special events, and academic or personal counselling (Keating, 2015). It is important to note that about one of every two undergraduate students at Canadian universities is taught by contract staff not generally involved in planning either the academic or the informal curricula at their institutions (Ellis-Hale, 2017).

In the health professions, curricula are profoundly influenced by the requirements of professional associations, regulatory bodies, and approval boards. Curricula must address discipline-specific competencies (Melrose, Park, & Perry, 2015). To achieve these competencies, partnerships with health-care agencies are usually required. In turn, agency structures exert influences on curricula. Furthermore, the "hidden" curricula (the customs, rituals, and taken-for-granted aspects of education in the health professions, particularly those that learners experience during interactions with faculty and clinicians in practice settings) also affect educational experiences (Hafferty, 1998; Hafferty & Franks, 1994; Hafferty & O'Donnell, 2014; Mahood, 2011).

Infusing the varied influences of academic, informal, and hidden curricula with humanity can make a substantial positive difference to pre-service and in-service learners in the health professions. For many learners, the memory of *how* a teacher brought a course outline or learning activity to life outlasts *what* the course required. In health professional education, many elements of the curriculum are mandated by professional associations and other governing bodies. At times, this required content can seem to be mundane and even uninspiring. The challenge for educators is to help learners see that knowledge of these elements becomes part of who they are as caring and competent practitioners. Students who acquire this required knowledge and come to know the governance and historical backdrops to their areas of practice are more fully prepared to provide comprehensive care experienced as humane. Educators skilled at infusing even the most tedious educational content with a sense of the human provide students with both knowledge (the what) and a positive sense of being taught by a humanizing educator (the how).

In this chapter, we begin by presenting a historical backdrop to illustrate how curricula in health professions education has evolved. We focus on the critical role that professional associations played in this transformation. Next, we discuss the influence of governance structures on curricula, introduce the

Tyler (1949) academic curriculum model, and provide a snapshot of aspects of informal and hidden curricula that can influence learners' experiences.

HISTORICAL BACKDROP

The philosophical underpinnings that guide curricula in specific health profession programs often evolved because of historical shifts and legacies that shaped higher education in general. These legacies can still be seen in academic curricula. Understanding connections with the past can help to clarify and evaluate present-day practices. In this section, we describe a select group of Canadian postsecondary educational and instructional practices at different times.

Service for Training

Health professionals were not always educated in universities. Many acquired their skills by providing services or unpaid work to organizations in return for an education. Known as "service for training," this historical curricular approach was common. In Canada, in the early 1900s, higher education consisted of only a small number of provincially funded universities and private denominational institutions. Many of these institutions relied on financial donations from patrons. Postsecondary educational institutions were not-for-profit organizations, served an elite fraction of the population, received only modest levels of provincial government funding, and operated with considerable autonomy (Jones, 2014). Each university had a unique University Act approved by the provincial legislature.

Physicians. University faculties included science, arts, theology, and only later medicine. Historically, education for physicians and other health professionals, including nurses, was provided by hospitals. Curricula were grounded in an apprenticeship model in which training was provided in return for service (Canadian Association of Schools of Nursing, 2012; Wytenbroek & Vandenberg, 2017).

In 1910, a landmark examination of medical schools in Canada and the United States, known as the Flexner Report, resulted in the closing of all hospital schools of medicine, and universities became responsible for the education of physicians (Flexner, 1910). Once physician education became integrated into university settings, schools of medicine shifted away from service for training approaches and embraced the scientific knowledge inherent in a biomedical curricular model (Duffy, 2011).

Nurses. Shifts away from service for training curricula did not come as readily for registered nurses (RNs) and other health professionals. Schools of nursing were housed in hospitals, which relied heavily on student nurses to provide care for patients. Curricula often revolved around staffing needs, and the educational needs of students inevitably took second place to hospital work-force requirements.

Hospital control over educational practices made it difficult to establish national standards for schools and their graduates (Pringle, Green, & Johnson, 2004). RN leaders began to look for opportunities to affiliate schools of nursing with Canadian universities as early as 1905, with the first baccalaureate degree program opening in 1919 (Canadian Association of Schools of Nursing, 2012).

However, hospital diploma programs were viewed as a fiscally prudent solution to ongoing nursing shortages and government funding deficits, and enrolments in hospital-based programs surged. In 1962, despite repeated efforts by professional organizations to integrate schools of nursing into universities, only 148 students graduated from baccalaureate degree programs, whereas 6,000 RNs graduated from hospital diploma programs (Canadian Association of Schools of Nursing, 2012).

A university education was not seen as a typical path for all nurses. Rather, the small group of nurses who attended university usually practised upon graduation in leadership roles, such as teaching or supervising, or worked in public health (Kirkwood, 2005). Teachers in hospital programs were referred to as instructors and generally held a baccalaureate degree. They were expected to be expert clinicians capable of sharing their hands-on knowledge and skills with learners.

Teachers in university programs were referred to as faculty and held a master's or doctoral degree. They were expected to engage in research. Although nursing students who attended universities were "educated," those in hospital programs were "trained." University communities often viewed nursing faculties as more suited to technical institutes, and in the 1970s there were too few faculty members to meet university standards for appointment (Pringle et al., 2004).

In 1965, a Royal Commission on Health Services report recommended that all nursing education come under the control of the educational institutions (Mussallem, 1965). This milestone report was instrumental in moving nursing education away from a service for training approach and toward university education as a requirement for entry to practice. The report recommended two categories of practitioner: professional nurses educated at universities and technical nurses educated in two-year college programs (Mussallem, 1965). Over the next three decades, hospital schools gradually moved into community college and university settings, with the last hospital-based programs closing in the 1990s (Dick & Cragg, 2003).

Professional nurses. To address the professional nurse category, universities offered basic and post-diploma programs so that both new and practising RNs from diploma programs could earn a baccalaureate degree in nursing (BN). By 2000, Canadian RNs were expected to hold a BN (Pringle et al., 2004). However, practice placements at hospitals and other clinical sites remained a critical element of university curricula. Therefore, though service for training had been eliminated, control over practicum placements remained with clinical agencies.

Technical nurses. To address the technical nurse category, programs for licensed practical nurses (LPNs)/registered practical nurses (RPNs) were created in vocational training sectors such as high schools, technical institutes, and hospitals. The title LPN is used mainly in western Canada, whereas the title RPN is used in eastern Canada. In other jurisdictions around the world, the title of vocational nurse (VN) or enrolled nurse (EN) is also used.

Programs for technical nurses were subject to top-down control from RN professional organizations or provincial/territorial ministries of health (Pringle et al., 2004). Early programs prepared graduates who would be "assistants" to RNs, and curricula were determined by RNs rather than LPNs/RPNs. Employing LPNs/RPNs rather than RNs was a cost-saving measure for health-care agencies, and in some instances they were viewed as replacements for hospital-trained RNs (Pringle et al., 2004).

By the 1990s, the Canadian Council for Practical Nurse Regulators, formerly the Canadian Practical Nurses Association, established an increased scope of practice, expanded curricula, and standardized examinations. Yet the legacy of "assisting" RNs rather than feeling as though they were "real nurses" persisted for LPNs/RPNs (Janzen, Melrose, Gordon, & Miller, 2013).

Overlapping scopes of practice between LPNs/RPNs and RNs created ambiguity and role confusion.

Limited collaboration. Limited collaboration existed among programs educating the two groups of nurses (RNs and LPNs/RPNs). Curricula in LPN/RPN programs were viewed as content driven, skills based, and geared to preparing job-ready nurses, whereas curricula in university programs were grounded in theories from nursing literature (Butcher, MacKinnon, & Bruce, 2018). Although universities such as Athabasca University, Canada's Open University, awarded transfer credits to LPNs/RPNs earning a BN (Athabasca University, n.d.), most universities required LPNs/RPNs to complete all BN program courses to earn a degree.

Organizational models attempted to ameliorate some of the tensions by differentiating among the responsibilities that nurses are expected to assume in the workplace. For example, one model, the Care Delivery Model Redesign, identified RN responsibilities as coordinating and providing care for the most acutely ill and unstable patients and LPN/RPN responsibilities as recognizing when patient outcomes are unpredictable and then transferring care to an RN (MacKinnon, Butcher, & Bruce, 2018). Even with these efforts, some role confusion remains in most workplaces.

Professional Associations

Historical shifts have contributed to influences on curricula for other health professionals as well as the physicians and nurses discussed above. Professional associations exerted significant influence on health professions curricula. Understanding how the professional associations evolved is an important aspect of learners' socialization into their professions. When educators share examples of how this evolution affected required knowledge, they can help learners to view that knowledge as stemming from real people who made a difference to their professions.

Social workers. As Jennissen and Lundy (2011) note, the education of Canadian social workers evolved over the past 80 years from brief periods of instruction supported by colleges of theology. Prior to the formation of the Canadian Association of Social Workers in 1926, Canadian social workers were members of American organizations and heavily influenced by political and social events occurring beyond Canada. The formation of a Canadian national professional organization created a foundation for standardizing social work curricula and practices among the provinces.

Physiotherapists. Initially educated under the auspices of medical schools, physiotherapists at one time were able to practise only in hospitals and under the direction of physicians (Fornasier, 2017). Early physiotherapists, most of whom were female nurses, were known as "reconstruction aides" for their work supporting injured First World War veterans to rebuild wasted muscles and use prosthetic limbs (Evans, 2010). Later, during the outbreak of polio in the 1920s, physiotherapists' groundbreaking use of massage and exercise treatments contributed to the treatment and rehabilitation of patients living with polio (Evans, 2010). In the 1950s, physiotherapy education moved away from medical schools and into independent schools of physiotherapy at universities (Fornasier, 2017).

Occupational therapists. Likewise, occupational therapists, known as "ward aides" in the 1920s, first practised under the direction of physicians in tuberculosis sanatoriums and mental hospitals (Prince Edward Island Occupational Therapy Society, n.d.). Early educational programs initiated in vocational training institutes in the 1930s later moved to universities in the 1950s and 1960s. As was the case with nurses, social workers, and physiotherapists, occupational therapists were slow to situate their education in universities. The formation of a Canadian national association helped occupational therapists to achieve standardized curricula and processes of accreditation and to become recognized as autonomous professionals (Prince Edward Island Occupational Therapy Society, n.d.).

Present-day academic curricula. Today many health professionals require university degrees at the entry to practice level. For example, RNs (Canadian Nurses Association, n.d.) and social workers (Canadian Association of Social Workers, n.d.) require a baccalaureate degree; physiotherapists (Canadian Physiotherapy Association, n.d.) and occupational therapists (Canadian Association of Occupational Therapists, n.d.) require a master's degree. Professional associations have played a key role in ensuring that opportunities for a university education are now available to most health professionals. Stories of how professional associations moved people who cared for the sick away from service for training models of instruction and into universities can shed new light on curricular activities in which learners are required to engage.

When educators invite learners to picture what a member of their profession might have looked like many decades ago, it can add a genuinely human element to information that might not seem to be immediately relevant.

In many instances, the current regulations, processes for approving programs, required curricula, and competencies expected of graduates imposed by professional associations have stemmed from past experiences of being subjugated by other professional groups or countries. Shifts away from service for training, the titles of assistant or ward aide, and the achievement of national standards did not come easily. Examining present-day academic curricula in relation to these shifts can provide valuable insights into why certain educational practices are valued more than others. Since most health professionals are now educated in universities, in addition to recognizing historical influences, it is important to consider how overarching university governance structures play a role in the instruction provided by specific programs. The strategy below can help educators to encourage learners to understand more about the historical backdrops that influenced their professions. Importantly, the activity reminds learners that real people (who had their own ideas, values, and beliefs) were the authors of the histories that comprise the foundations of their disciplines.

A STRATEGY TO TRY

"Old School" Stories

Invite experienced colleagues to share old school stories about their education. Open conversations with questions such as "what stands out for you when you think back on your education?" and "can you tell me about practices that seem different now from when you were learning?" As you enjoy and appreciate the stories, notice how external factors (i.e., factors beyond specific programs) affect the educational experience. For example, did staffing or funding issues related to a clinical agency influence the academic curriculum?

If you find this strategy useful, then create opportunities during practicums in which learners can invite clinicians to share old school stories about their education.

As the previous discussion illustrated, institutions that provided educational programs for health professionals, whether they were hospitals, universities, or other postsecondary institutions, exerted significant control over curricula. Governance structures dictated how institutions were financed and managed. In turn, these structures (and the people who worked and learned in them) affected specific programs. Next, we provide a brief overview of key governance structures common to most Canadian universities.

Bicameral Governance

Historically, postsecondary institutions, particularly universities, were governed under a bicameral structure in which the responsibility for administrative and fiscal matters was assigned to a governing board and the responsibility for academic matters was assigned to a senate or academic council (Jones, Shanahan, & Goyan, 2004). Governing board members were usually external to the university and appointed by the provincial government, whereas senates were largely composed of a select group of internal members such as academic administrators and senior faculty (Jones, 2014). The bicameral structure afforded external accountability and provided clarification of the separate responsibilities expected in university-government relationships (Jones et al., 2004).

After the Second World War, mainly during the 1960s and 1970s, systems of higher education, which included both university and non-university postsecondary sectors, expanded from an elite to a mass system as more and more people expected to obtain an education that extended beyond high school (Jones, 2013). In response to swelling enrolments at universities, provincial funding was supplemented by transfer payments from the federal government, though the provinces retained control of postsecondary institutions.

As individual postsecondary institutions became increasingly more dependent on government funding, their autonomy eroded significantly. Curricula in all programs were affected by funding decisions. Provincial governments increased their involvement in the institutions that they funded, resulting in frequent conflicts. Boundaries between responsibilities that politicians could undertake and those previously assumed by institutional leaders were seldom clear (Jones, 2014). Universities were no longer the not-for-profit institutions attended by the privileged few as they once were.

Accountability for public funding, and demands for more inclusive governance, led to lasting reforms of the bicameral board/senate model. The Duff-Berdahl Report called for more faculty, student, and community representation on university boards and senates (Duff & Berdahl, 1966). To increase openness and transparency, interaction and communication between boards and senates increased, and meetings previously held behind closed doors were opened to public observation (Jones, 2014). Since the 1970s, most Canadian institutions have continued to be governed by this reformed bicameral model.

Faculty Employment

Over the past five decades, mass attendance, governance reforms, and public accountability, particularly during times of economic downturn, also led to changes in the employment of postsecondary teachers. Faculty are employed either in full-time continuing positions or in part-time contract positions. At universities, full-time faculty are expected to engage in a combination of research, teaching, and service activities (Jones, 2014). For many full-time faculty, maintaining a robust program of research and publication accomplishments leaves limited time for creating teaching innovations or participating in curriculum planning. In turn, the critical tasks of developing, revising, and evaluating curricula might be done by only a small group of faculty members. If the team tasked with curriculum development or revision embraces the value of creating a humanizing curriculum, then the outcome can be courses and programs focused in this way. Alternatively, because in reality only a few faculty members usually undertake curriculum development/redevelopment, if they are limited in their humanizing focus, then the outcome can be an educational experience void of a focus on the humane.

Funding issues continue to dominate employment practices at postsecondary institutions. Labour cost efficiencies have been created by increasing the use of part-time contract teachers (Jones, 2013). It is estimated that more than half of all undergraduates at Canadian universities are taught by part-time contract faculty (Basen, 2014; Ellis-Hale, 2017).

Over the past decade, contract faculty have become the new majority at universities (Fitzpatrick, 2017; Gappa, 2008; Meixner, Kruck, & Madden, 2010). Part-time faculty contracts can offer positions such as limited-term full-time faculty (Rajagopal, 2004), part-time faculty, sessional instructors, term instructors (Puplampu, 2004), and adjunct faculty (Meixner et al., 2010).

Many of these faculty "are paid per course taught and are seldom offered benefits such as health insurance or access to retirement plans" (Meixner et al., 2010, p. 141).

The trend toward employing short-term contract faculty "spotlights a new norm of precarious labor in academia" (Fitzpatrick, 2017, para. 2). At many institutions, part-time contractual and full-time continuing faculty are members of separate unions (Jones, 2014). Part-time contract faculty generally have limited opportunities to develop and evaluate the curricula that they deliver. In some sense, when individuals are unsure of how committed the organization is to them as real people with individual needs, likes, and priorities, they can experience their workplaces as dehumanizing. Creating a humanizing workplace is foundational to inspiring educators (and subsequently learners) to practise humanely.

Balancing Multiple Governance Structures

In Canada today, most universities are secular institutions reliant on provincial funding, though small private universities, often associated with a religious denomination, are allowed in some provinces (Jones, 2014). Other postsecondary institutions include public and private colleges as well as technical/vocational institutes. Programs for health professionals are offered at most of these different institutions, and students often transition between sectors.

Additionally, clinical agencies and professional associations offer staff development, continuing education, and certification programs, usually for in-service learners. Not unexpectedly, the structures governing individual institutions in each sector are very different. Infusing curricula with humanity while balancing the requirements of multiple governance structures poses a unique challenge to educators of health professionals.

Student attendance at multiple institutions requires educators in health profession programs to comply with a range of administrative and fiscal governance structures. Universities and clinical agencies have separate systems for governance and regulation. For example, at universities, where funding is dependent on provincial governments, politicians can determine that funding for a program will be reduced. Because staffing decisions are made by governing boards, a board of governors can require more part-time than full-time employment of faculty. A university senate committee, with responsibilities for academic matters, can provide input into practicum courses even when members of the committee are not health professionals.

Furthermore, the clinical agencies at which students complete required practicums are governed by health-care boards. Issues of patient/client safety, capacity to integrate learners, and funding cuts dictate the extent to which boards can support health profession programs. The structures governing the many different institutions where health professionals learn play important roles in the specific programs offered. In the next section, we provide an overview of a common curricular model frequently used to guide educational and instructional practices. Before reading about this model, consider ways in which you can find out more about the governance model at your institution. How does governance structure affect curricula and how you work with learners? The strategy below suggests a way to view governance structures as simply being a group of people.

A STRATEGY TO TRY

Put Faces to Names

Investigate the governance model at the institution where you teach or would like to teach. Try to put faces to the names of people in leadership positions. In postsecondary settings, is the institution governed under a board/senate bicameral structure in which administrative and fiscal matters are managed by a governing board and academic matters are managed by a senate or academic council? In clinical agency settings, how are the institutions governed? What are the sources of funding? How do funding decisions affect your day-to-day work with learners? Can you get a sense of the nature of the governance approach or the environment created by administrators in this organization? Are there any clues to whether the approach and environment are humanizing or dehumanizing?

How can you become involved and learn more about governance? For example, can you attend board/senate meetings as an observer? Are there opportunities to contribute your feedback and ideas either individually or as a member of a committee? The process can begin by simply getting to know the names of members of governing boards/ senates and then putting faces to those names. Understanding governance relationships can begin like understanding any other human

> relationship . . . by reaching out and getting to know the people involved.

THE TYLER ACADEMIC CURRICULUM MODEL

Curricula can be viewed as the plans or roadmaps that guide student learning. In academic or formal learning settings, curricular models can be used to represent activities expected of educators and learners. These models can be used to map activities at program, course, and even individual levels. Most programs make overarching outcomes expected of graduates available to the public; study guides or course outlines available to students and faculty involved in the course; and individual orientation/assessment activities available to the faculty, students, and clinicians participating in them. Curricula (especially in health professions in which there are continuous changes to elements such as medications, treatments, and procedures) are dynamic and require ongoing development, evaluation, and revision.

Various curricular models are implemented in programs educating health professionals. Iwasiw, Andrusyszyn, and Goldenberg (2018) emphasize the importance of evidence, context, and unity in any model of curriculum development. Neville-Norton and Cantwell (2019) highlight the value of collaboration and collective dialogue among faculty throughout the process of designing and delivering curricula. A full description of the complexities inherent in understanding and applying models to develop, evaluate, and revise curricula is beyond the scope of this chapter. Rather, we provide a brief introduction to the classic Tyler Model, which has guided educators in creating curricula in both general and health profession programs since the 1950s (Meek, 1993; Tyler, 1949). Clearly, there are many potential links between the curricular model endorsed by an educational institution and the nature of the curriculum designed. The model used helps educators designing courses and programs to make decisions about what is taught and how educators interact with learners. A more human-focused model should bring about a more humanizing curriculum.

The Tyler Model has been criticized for presenting a prescriptive, linear, and objective-centred approach that neglects the cyclical and constantly evolving nature of curricula (Hlebowitsh, 1992, 1995; Kliebard, 1970, 1995). Critical thinking, problem solving, and professional values can be difficult to articulate into behavioural objectives that can be measured. However, under-standing the underlying principles of teaching that frame the model provides important and enduring guidance for educators in competency-based health profession programs (Cruickshank, 2018; Wraga, 2017).

Tyler (1949) identified four critical teaching principles to consider when creating curricula. First, *determine the purpose or objectives of the program/course/individual activity*. This principle requires educators to consider what learners need, and what they must do, in order to be successful. Standards and competencies required by educational institutions, professional associations, and national licensing boards must always be considered. The purpose of activities in programs or courses is also expected to be consistent with the needs of society in general. In health professions education, public safety is a critical factor in planning learning experiences, particularly those in which novice students/practitioners provide care to patients/clients. Furthermore, the purpose of all activities should be consistent with the philosophy of the school or discipline. In other words, links between learning activities and necessary disciplinary knowledge should be clear. As educators and learners work collaboratively through curricula, the purpose of the activities that they engage in should clarify both the behaviour or competency to be developed and the content to be applied.

Second, *provide useful educational experiences to support that purpose*. This principle calls educators to examine the design and content of educational activities in relation to the purpose of the program/course/activity. Context-ual factors play important roles in providing useful educational experiences. For example, clinical practice opportunities differ between rural and urban areas. Some learners might not have access to pre-clinical skill labs and simu-lation equipment. Non-traditional clinical placements (e.g., at shelters for the homeless) might or might not align with course objectives designed for traditional clinical agency placements such as hospital units. Specific prepar-ations for national licensing exams might be useful educational experiences that planners of curricula had not previously considered. Taking these and other contextual factors into consideration, the importance of educators and learners continuing to question whether an experience is useful, not useful, or in need of evaluation becomes clear.

Third, *organize learning experiences to have a maximum cumulative effect*. Here imposing a logical order on the content presented and the experiences in which learners participate is important. Individual learning activities should be organized in ways that demonstrate continuity, sequence, and integration into the courses and programs with which they are associated. Content and learning activities during the early stages of courses and programs should be less complex than at the later stages. Once again, the unique nature of education in the health professions poses challenges when providing activities that progress from less difficult to more difficult, especially in clinical courses. High-acuity clinical agencies limit educators' ability to scaffold experiences in which learners first care for stable patients and then later, as their knowledge and confidence increase, provide care to very ill patients. In essence, this principle casts a spotlight on the importance of understanding student learning beyond activities in a specific course.

Fourth, *evaluate curricula and revise ineffective aspects.* Tyler's (1949) model was designed to measure the degree to which predefined objectives and outcomes were attained. Therefore, this teaching principle involves the complex process of evaluating individual students' learning as well as the curricular experiences with which they were provided. For example, information that students completed a learning activity and were able attain an objective would contribute to evaluation of their curriculum. Alternatively, information that some students were not able to attain an objective also contributes to evaluation of their curriculum. In this instance, part of the evaluation includes further investigation. Questions must be asked about the adequacy of the learning experiences provided, the individual student's participation in those learning activities, the degree to which other students were/were not able to attain the same objective, and the methods of evaluation implemented to measure the degree to which the student was able/unable to attain the objective. In turn, these questions open the door to discussions about curricular revisions.

Although at first glance the Tyler Model might not seem to be especially compatible with deriving a humanity-focused curriculum, some elements of the model do aid in this outcome. For example, there is a focus on individual student learning. This is a recognition that each person is unique and might obtain learning outcomes at a pace or in a way unlike other learners. This recognition of individuality is humanizing. Tyler (1949) also emphasizes the humanizing principle of collaboration, working together respectfully to attain more than any one person could attain alone. The respect essential in true collaboration is predicated on a level of trust within relationships among collaborators. Trust is also essential in acting humanely. Finally, Tyler recognized the importance of context. Human lives are embedded in unique contexts, and recognizing the roles of context in lives, relationships, actions, and interactions is essential to behaving humanely.

Determining whether an aspect of a curriculum is ineffective and in need of revision is seldom straightforward. Inclusive, collaborative, and ongoing discussions among all of the educators and clinicians who teach students are necessary. Facilitating these discussions can be difficult when educators work in different academic or clinical institutions and have employment contracts that do not include curricular planning. The strategy below might be a useful starting point if you are considering evaluation and possible revision of a curriculum. It also provides a means to include student voices in this process, essential to forging a curriculum that embraces the value of all participants.

A Strategy to Try

Why Are We Doing This?

Select a learning activity in which learners with whom you are familiar participate. Apply the four teaching principles espoused in the Tyler Model to this activity. The learners can be pre-service or in-service students whom you teach at a university or precept in your workplace. The learning activity can be completed in face-to-face classrooms, online classrooms, or clinical practicums. It can be completed in a group or individually as a self-study. To apply the model, answer the following questions.

1. What is the *purpose* of the activity? What is the behaviour or competency to be developed, and what is the content to be applied? Is the link between this activity and disciplinary knowledge clear?

2. Is this activity the best and most *useful* way to acquire this disciplinary knowledge?

3. Where does this activity fit in relation to the *organization* of other activities in the course or program?

4. Does this activity do what it was designed to do? Does it support learners in successfully demonstrating competencies? Which

> processes are or could be in place to communicate your evaluation
> of and suggested *revisions* to the activity?

Educators' and learners' experiences with curricula are not limited to those outlined by academics through models such as the Tyler Model. Less formal activities also make significant contributions to what, and how, students learn. In the next section, we provide a brief overview of how informal curricula can influence learning in the health professions.

INFORMAL CURRICULA

Beyond the structured academic curricula that guide classroom and clinical practicum courses, students in the health professions are also influenced by informal curricular experiences that can contribute to their learning. Depending on institutional capacity, these informal experiences can include opportunities to interact with faculty and fellow learners, support/counselling services or help centres, sport and fitness programs, religious/cultural gathering places, and children's daycare, to name just a few. Unfortunately, clinical agency requirements and busy schedules can limit participation in some of these experiences.

Clinical agency requirements in off-campus practicum courses include early morning, evening, and weekend shifts, making it difficult for learners to take advantage of support services and participate regularly in extracurricular activities. Clinical agencies are often unable to accommodate student requests for changes to the days or times that they are scheduled to attend their placement sessions. Learners must be supervised by clinical instructors or preceptors, and most clinical sites host students from multiple programs, so placement spaces are restricted and often scarce. This can greatly affect whether or not students experience their practice learning experiences as humane.

Hectic schedules sway students' thinking in relation to informal curricula that they perceive as optional. Learners in health profession programs include both traditional and non-traditional students. Traditional students are those who recently graduated from high school. Non-traditional students, also referred to as mature students or adult learners, are over 25 years of age. They might have one or more of the following characteristics: they have delayed their postsecondary enrolment or are returning to their studies, have one or more dependants, attend school part time, and/or are employed full time (Ross-Gordon, 2011).

Since 1996, nearly 70% of all undergraduate students also possess at least one non-traditional characteristic (National Center for Education Statistics, 2015). Academic demands, full schedules, and family/employment commitments can limit the time that students spend engaging in activities not directly related to program requirements. However, two key areas of informal curricula are of particular relevance to health profession students: opportunities to interact with faculty and fellow students and support services for language learning. These elements of the informal curricula are often the essentials that humanize learning experiences for students.

Opportunities to Interact with Faculty and Students

Times when students can informally interact and connect with their teachers and one another can bring content to life in new and exciting ways. Interpersonal relationships between students and their teachers are highly valued (Collier, 2018). These relationships create opportunities in which educators can reveal their own processes of thinking critically, and they allow educators to model problem-solving approaches (Raymond, Profetto-McGrath, Myrick, & Strean, 2018). Similarly, peer relationships have been shown to develop students' skills in communication, critical thinking, and self-confidence (Stone, Cooper, & Cant, 2013).

Despite their value, opportunities for informal interactions to occur among faculty and students can be overshadowed by the demands of academic curricula. Faculty schedules, like student schedules, are often hectic. Teaching in multiple institutional and clinical settings can leave faculty with only limited time for impromptu hallway conversations, after-class question-answer sessions, pre-/post-assignment discussions, and bedside patient/client debriefing reviews with individual students.

Part-time employment categories can stipulate the times when, places where, and planned activities in which contact with students occurs. Full-time faculty committed to research projects might have fewer teaching responsibilities, leaving them with infrequent opportunities to interact with students. When clinicians interact with students, their priority must always be their patients/clients, and interruptions during conversations with learners happen frequently as clinicians are called away to provide patient/client care.

Educational institutions can implement student success centres in which call centre models respond to common student questions and concerns. Such centres were initially developed to improve student persistence and program completion, but there is considerable variation in how they are managed across educational sectors and by individual institutions (Smith, Baldwin, & Schmidt, 2015). For institutions that implement call centre models, teaching time can be managed efficiently, and responses to students can be expected to be prompt, consistent, and accurate. Nevertheless, once student callers have answers to their questions, further dialogue and spontaneous conversation (which can be humanizing) are unlikely.

Peer interactions often occur naturally among students before, during, and after shared learning experiences. Gathering spaces where students can come together to debrief activities, form study groups, and share strategies are an important aspect of informal curricula that should be cultivated. When physical spaces in educational institutions or clinical facilities are not available, students can meet at nearby coffee shops or on video conferencing call programs. In online settings, students also value having gathering spaces in which they can discuss common interests and support one another (Melrose, Moore, & Ewing, 2013). Creating spaces for informal peer interaction, and encouraging learners to use them fully, can easily infuse humanity into curricula. The following idea emphasizes the importance of creating opportunities for interactions with students by establishing office hours.

A STRATEGY TO TRY

My Office Hours Are . . .

In most educational settings, the term "office hours" is a recognizable expression of specific times when teachers make themselves available to students. Traditionally, appointment times were posted on office doors. Today online scheduling programs, web conferencing, and interactive learning platforms provide a range of opportunities for educators to post office hours.

Pre-service and in-service learners alike need unstructured time in which they can initiate conversations, explore ideas, and begin to form interpersonal connections with faculty, instructors, preceptors, and clinicians involved in their programs. When you meet learners in your teaching practice, which tools of communication can you implement to inform them of your office hours? How will you complete the sentence "my office hours are. . . ."

Language Learning Support

Another key area of informal curricula relevant to health professions education is language learner support. Like most students in developed countries, Canadian postsecondary students come from a variety of educational and socio-cultural backgrounds with as many as 22% needing explicit support with language learning (Brancato, 2016). In health professions education in predominantly English-speaking areas of Canada, challenges that many English as a Second Language (ESL) students face include difficulty communicating effectively with patients in English, inability to succeed academically throughout their programs, and struggling to pass national licensing exams (Choi, 2005, 2016).

Learners are expected to be proficient in the language used by the institution that they are attending, whether it confers degrees, diplomas, certificates, or continuing education credits. When institutions have the capacity to provide services for language support, it is essential to ensure that students who need them have opportunities to access them. When institutions do not provide this support, explore other resources in the community that learners can access. The strategy below suggests how you could achieve this.

A STRATEGY TO TRY

Where Are Language Support Services?

Locate language support services available to learners with whom you are involved. These services might be provided at a learning institution, a clinical agency, or in the community. They might be offered in face-to-face or online settings and be provided to groups and/or individuals. How easy or difficult are they to access? How can you help learners who need these services to initiate and maintain contact? Is there a need to advocate for additional services relevant to learners in the health professions? In the absence of language support services, can you initiate study groups in which learners who need help can receive (and provide) peer assistance or share resources with one another?

Implicit Messages

Hidden curricula are the implicit messages about values, norms, and attitudes that learners infer from the role models and structures that they observe around them (Hafferty & Franks, 1994). Educators do not intend to communicate these messages, and they are often unaware of their existence (Cowell, 1972). Dewey (1938) used the term "collateral learning" to describe hidden curricula.

At the institutional/organizational, interpersonal/social, contextual/cultural, and motivational/psychological levels, these implicit messages shape how learners make sense of the environments that surround their learning (Lawrence et al., 2018). When institutions fund some programs but not others, when educators spend time discussing a specific topic, when clinicians pay attention to a particular condition/illness, and when a certain behaviour is acknowledged with awards or promotions, learners inherently draw conclusions about the highly valued aspects of their profession.

Similarly, vision and mission statements might espouse a value, but ways of speaking or "institutional slang" used at the institution can suggest that the value does not translate fully into practice (Hafferty, 1998). As Semper and Blasco (2018, p. 11) emphasize, transmitting values important to disciplines, institutions, and programs through explicit official documents such as statements on mission, vision, and values is incomplete "because it is the teacher who teaches, not the official documents." Educators are essential in helping learners to understand and internalize the visions and missions of the organizations in which they study and practise and in guiding students to enact the associated values.

Logically, when implicit messages, rewarded behaviours, and organizations' missions, visions, and values are humanizing (or promote the humane), all participants are made aware that these types of relationships are the goal and valued more highly. To create a humanizing educational institution, program, or curriculum, the first step might be to infuse the hidden curricula with the same elements.

Parallel Education

As learners begin their programs, they receive what Chen (2015, p. 7) refers to as a "parallel education in professional socialization" through hidden curricula. Their parallel education or hidden curricula "does not *explicitly* dismiss or contradict the formal . . . curriculum. Rather, it runs subtly alongside or underneath the formal curriculum, and permeates its interstitial spaces" (p. 8). As Chen notes, hidden curricula vary from discipline to discipline and among programs, depending on the history, culture, structure, and practices that have evolved. A common denominator is that what educators and clinicians *do* can exert more influence than what they *say*.

Adapting the implicit messages inherent in parallel or hidden curricula, many of which are negative, outdated, and even unjust, into tools that can support learning is not easy. Without intentionally addressing these implicit messages, their influence can dilute content presented in planned curricula. When educators in classrooms present a theoretical position, but that position is not reflected in the actions and practices of learners in their interactions with educators and clinicians, it is likely to be disregarded. Making implicit messages more explicit begins with acknowledging them (Chen, 2015; Semper & Blasco, 2018).

Instead of ignoring or denying hidden curricula, when educators acknowledge the inadvertent and often conflicting messages that learners experience, they communicate a willingness to engage in further conversations. Chen (2015) asserted that the purpose of acknowledging and talking about the hidden curriculum is neither to eradicate it nor to create more content for lectures and other learning activities in formal academic curricula.

Sensitive, open discussions when learners feel conflicted provide occasions for educators and clinicians to share their own experiences and processes of working through issues. Such an approach can be experienced by all as respectful of their unique humanity. These discussions tap into the parallel education that is occurring and offer opportunities for educators to model critical thinking. As Chen wrote,

> when we address messages in the hidden curriculum with moral imagination and practical wisdom, students tune in; they observe our approaches to situations that arise, and how we respond. This gives us an opportunity

to play a positive role in the formation of students' professional identity. Modelling these behaviours for our students helps them to develop and internalize a nuanced approach to professional practice. (2015, p. 14)

Taking opportunities that arise to discuss aspects of the hidden curricula can provide educators with openings to share their humanity with learners.

Making implicit curricula more explicit does not mean that educators are expected to have all the answers. Just as learners are continually piecing together messages from people with whom they interact in their classrooms and practicum sites, so too educators are sorting through messages from their professional associations, employment contracts, and governance structures at multiple sites.

To serve as meaningful role models to students, educators must also acknowledge that hidden messages exist and engage in open discussions about their impacts. Perhaps most importantly, educators must maintain an ongoing process of self-questioning about how they might contribute to and perpetuate negative values, norms, and attitudes. Shedding light on hidden curricula is not a one-way transmission of insight and wisdom from educators to learners. Rather, it is a dialogue rooted in curiosity, personal perceptions, and shared reasoning. And what could be more humane or a greater factor in promoting humanity than sensitive, other-focused, attentive dialogue?

CONCLUSION

In this chapter, we explored ways of infusing curricula with humanity. Like roadmaps, curricula provide predetermined structures to guide educators and learners. Curricula in health professional education often reflect connections to the past. To illustrate this connection, we offered a snapshot of Canadian postsecondary educational and instructional practices at different points in time. Professional associations have played key roles in establishing national standards and making opportunities for a university education available, and they continue to exert significant influence on the competencies expected of practitioners.

Pre-service and in-service learners in the health professions access educational activities from a variety of organizations. Programs and learning experiences can be provided at universities, other postsecondary institutions such as colleges or technical institutes, and clinical agencies. Governance of these organizations, particularly control of finances and management, also exerts influence on curricula. Furthermore, employment contracts can stipulate the nature of contact between educators and learners. Governance structures can restrict opportunities for educators and clinicians to collaborate on developing, evaluating, and revising curricula. Despite these restrictions, when educators make efforts to reach out to colleagues and learners, they can find ways to begin establishing the human connections so essential to bringing curricula to life.

One model of academic curricula, the Tyler Model (Tyler 1949), highlights four teaching principles that educators can apply to support learners in achieving required competencies. With any learning activity, course, or program, the principles can be summarized with the following questions. What is the purpose? Is this the most useful approach to attain this purpose? Where does it fit within the organization of other activities? Which revisions are needed?

Finally, we commented on how informal and hidden curricula also influence learning experiences. Beyond the program outcomes and course syllabus structures commonly planned in academic curricula, informal structures, such as designated spaces where learners can interact with educators and one another, and access to language learning supports for those who need them must also be considered. Hidden curricula affect professional socialization, and educators and clinicians must remain vigilant in examining whether what they *say* actually matches what they *do*. The heart of meaningful curricula— whether academic, informal, or hidden—is the essential human connection between educators and learners. Conversations with faculty, peers, and clinicians create lasting and impactful memories for learners.

REFERENCES

Athabasca University. (n.d.). *Post-LPN Bachelor of Nursing*. Retrieved from http://www.athabascau.ca/programs/summary/post-lpn-bachelor-of-nursing/

Basen, I. (2014, September 7). Most university undergrads now taught by poorly paid part-timers. *CBC News*. Retrieved from http://www.cbc.ca/news/canada/most-university-undergrads-now-taught-by-poorly-paid-part-timers-1.2756024

Brancato, E. (2016). *English language learners (ELL) undergraduate program development at OCAD University: Needs assessment summary and recommendations*. Toronto, ON: Ontario College of Art and Design.

Butcher, D., MacKinnon, K., & Bruce, A. (2018). Producing flexible nurses: How institutional texts organize nurses' experiences of learning to work on redesigned nursing teams. *Quality Advancement in Nursing Education, 4*(2), Article 2. doi:10.17483/2368-6669.1132

Canadian Association of Occupational Therapists. (n.d.). *Becoming an occupational therapist.* Retrieved from https://www.caot.ca/site/rfs/res_for_ students?nav=sidebar

Canadian Association of Schools of Nursing. (2012). *Ties that bind: The evolution of education for professional nursing in Canada from the 17th to the 21st century.* Ottawa, ON: Author. Retrieved from https://www.casn.ca/wp-content/ uploads/2016/12/History.pdf

Canadian Association of Social Workers. (n.d.). *How do I become a social worker?* Retrieved from https://www.casw-acts.ca/en/what-social-work/how-do-i- become-social-worker

Canadian Nurses Association. (n.d.). *Becoming an RN.* Retrieved from https://www. cna-aiic.ca/en/nursing-practice/the-practice-of-nursing/becoming-an-rn

Canadian Physiotherapy Association. (n.d.). *Become a PT or PTA.* Retrieved from https://physiotherapy.ca/becoming-pt-or-pta

Chen, R. (2015). Do as we say or do as we do? Examining the hidden curriculum in nursing education. *Canadian Journal of Nursing Research, 47*(3), 7–17. doi:10.1177/084456211504700301

Choi, L. (2005). Literature review: Issues surrounding education of English-as-a- Second Language (ESL) nursing students. *Journal of Transcultural Nursing, 16*(3), 263–268. doi:10.1177/1043659605274966

Choi, L. S. (2016). A support program for English as an additional language nursing students. *Journal of Transcultural Nursing, 27*(1), 81–85. doi:10.1177/1043659614554014

Collier, A. (2018). Characteristics of an effective nursing clinical instructor: The state of the science. *Journal of Clinical Nursing, 27,* 363–374. doi:10.1111/jocn.13931

Cowell, R. N. (1972). *The hidden curriculum: A theoretical framework and a pilot study.* Cambridge, MA: Harvard Graduate School of Education.

Cruickshank, V. (2018). Considering Tyler's curriculum model in health and physical education. *Journal of Education and Educational Development, 5*(1), 207–214. Retrieved from https://files.eric.ed.gov/fulltext/EJ1180613.pdf

Dewey, J. (1938). *Experience and education.* Indianapolis, IN: Free Press.

Dick, D. D., & Cragg, B. (2003). Undergraduate education: Development and politics. In M. McIntyre & E. Thomlinson (Eds.), *Realities of Canadian nursing* (p. 182–204). Philadelphia, PA: Lippincott Williams & Wilkins.

Duff, J., & Berdahl, R. (1966). *University government in Canada.* Ottawa, ON: Association of Universities and Colleges of Canada and Canadian Association of University Teachers.

Duffy, T. (2011). The Flexner Report—100 years later. *Yale Journal of Biology and Medicine, 84*(3), 269–276. Retrieved from https://www.ncbi.nlm.nih.gov/pmc/articles/PMC3178858/

Egan, K. (1978). What is curriculum? *Journal for the Canadian Association for Curriculum Studies, 9*(1), 9–16. Retrieved from https://jcacs.journals.yorku.ca/index.php/jcacs/article/viewFile/16845/15651

Egan, K. (2003). What is curriculum? *Curriculum Inquiry, 8*(1), 65–72. doi:10.1080/0 3626784.1978.11075558

Ellis-Hale, K. (2017). By the numbers: Contract academic staff in Canada. *Canadian Association of University Teachers Bulletin, 10*. Retrieved from https://www.caut.ca/bulletin/2017/10/numbers-contract-academic-staff-canada

Evans, S. (2010). Coming in the front door: A history of three Canadian physiotherapists through two world wars. *Canadian Military History, 19*(2), Article 5. http://scholars.wlu.ca/cmh/vol19/iss2/5

Fitzpatrick, M. (2017, October 22). Ontario college strike spotlights "new norm" of precarious labour in academia. *CBC News*. Retrieved from https://www.cbc.ca/news/canada/ontario-college-strike-academia-1.4364735

Flexner, A. (1910). *Medical education in the United Sates and Canada*. Washington, DC: Science and Health Publications.

Fornasier, R. (2017). A century-long struggle towards professionalism: Key factors in the growth of the physiotherapists' role in the United States, from subordinated practitioners to autonomous professionals. *Management and Organizational History, 12*(2), 142–162. doi:10.1080/17449359.2017.1329090

Gappa, J. M. (2008). Today's majority: Faculty outside the tenure system. *Change: The Magazine of Higher Learning, 40*(4), 50–54. doi:10.3200/CHNG.40.4.50-54

Hafferty, F. (1998). Beyond curriculum reform: Confronting medicine's hidden curriculum. *Academic Medicine, 73*(4), 403–407.

Hafferty, F., & Franks, R. (1994). The hidden curriculum, ethics teaching, and the structure of medical education. *Academic Medicine, 69*(11), 861–871.

Hafferty, F., & O'Donnell, J. (Eds.). (2014). *The hidden curriculum in health professional education*. Hanover, NH: Dartmouth College Press.

Hlebowitsh, P. (1992). Amid behavioural and behaviouristic objectives: Reappraising appraisals of the Tyler rationale. *Journal of Curriculum Studies, 24*(6), 533–547.

Hlebowitsh, P. (1995). Interpretations of the Tyler rationale: A reply to Kliebard. *Journal of Curriculum Studies, 27*(1), 89–94.

Iwasiw, C., Andrusyszyn, M., & Goldenberg, D. (2018). *Curriculum development in nursing education* (4th ed). Burlington, MA: Jones & Bartlett Learning.

Janzen, K., Melrose, S., Gordon, K., & Miller, J. (2013). "RN means real nurse": Perceptions of being a "real" nurse in a post-LPN-BN bridging program. *Nursing Forum, 48*(3), 165–73. doi:10.1111/nuf.12026

Jennissen, T., & Lundy, C. (2011). *One hundred years of social work: A history of the profession in English Canada*. Waterloo, ON: Wilfrid Laurier University Press.

Jones, G. (2013). The horizontal and vertical fragmentation of academic work and the challenge for academic governance and leadership. *Pacific Education Review, 14*(1), 75–83. Retrieved from https://tspace.library.utoronto.ca/bitstream/1807/43775/1/G%20Jones%20Horizontal-Vertical%20Academic%20Work.pdf

Jones, G. (2014). An introduction to higher education in Canada. In K. M. Joshi and S. Paivandi (Eds.), *Higher education across nations* (Vol. 1, p. 1–38). Delhi, India: B. R. Publishing. Retrieved from https://www.researchgate.net/publication/268512684_An_Introduction_to_Higher_Education_in_Canada

Jones, G., Shanahan, T., & Goyan, P. (2004). The academic senate and university governance in Canada. *The Canadian Journal of Higher Education, 34*(2), 35–68. Retrieved from http://journals.sfu.ca/cjhe/index.php/cjhe/article/viewFile/183456/183409

Jung, C. G. (2014). *The collected works of C.G. Jung: Complete digital edition*. Princeton, N.J.: Princeton University Press.

Keating, S. (2015). *Curriculum development and evaluation in nursing* (3rd ed.). New York, NY: Springer.

Kirkwood, L. (2005). Enough but not too much: Nursing education in English language Canada (1874–2000). In C. Bates, D. Dodd, & N. Rousseau (Eds.), *On all frontiers: Four centuries of Canadian nursing* (p. 183–196). Ottawa, ON: University of Ottawa Press.

Kliebard, H. M. (1970). Reappraisal: The Tyler rationale. *School Review, 78*, 259–272.

Kliebard, H. M. (1995). The Tyler rationale revisited. *Journal of Curriculum Studies, 27*(1), 81–88.

Lawrence, C., Mhlaba, T., Stewart, K, Moletsane, R., Gaede, B., & Moshabela, M. (2018). The hidden curricula of medical education: A scoping review. *Academic Medicine, 93*(4), 648–656. doi:10.1097/ACM.0000000000002004

MacKinnon, K., Butcher, D., & Bruce, A. (2018). Working to full scope: The reorganization of nursing work in two Canadian community hospitals. *Global Qualitative Nursing Research, 5*, 1–4. doi:10.1177/2333393617753390

Mahood, S. C. (2011). Medical education: Beware the hidden curriculum. *Canadian Family Physician, 57*(9), 983–985. Retrieved from https://www.ncbi.nlm.nih.gov/pmc/articles/PMC3173411/

Meek, A. (1993). On setting the highest standards: A conversation with Ralph Tyler. *Educational Leadership, 50*, 83–86. Retrieved from http://www.ascd.org/publications/educational-leadership/mar93/vol50/num06/On-Setting-the-Highest-Standards@-A-Conversation-with-Ralph-Tyler.aspx

Meixner, C., Kruck, S. E., & Madden, L. T. (2010). Inclusion of part-time faculty for the benefit of faculty and students. *College Teaching, 58*, 141–147.

Melrose, S., Moore, S., & Ewing, H. (2013). Chapter 5: Online interest groups for graduate students: Benefit or burden? In V. Wang (Ed.), *Advanced research in adult learning and professional development: Tools, trends, and methodologies*, 121–132. Hershey, PA: IGI Global.

Melrose, S., Park, C., & Perry, B. (2015). *Creative clinical teaching in the health professions.* Retrieved from http://epub-fhd.athabascau.ca/clinical-teaching/

Mussallem, H. K. (1965). *Nursing education in Canada.* (Submission to the Royal Commission on Health Services). Ottawa, ON: Queen's Printer.

National Center for Education Statistics. (2015). *Demographic and enrollment characteristics of nontraditional undergraduates: 2011–12.* Retrieved from https://nces.ed.gov/pubs2015/2015025.pdf

Neville-Norton, M., & Cantwell, S. (2019). Curriculum mapping in nursing education: A case study for collaborative curriculum design and program quality assurance. *Teaching and Learning in Nursing, 14*, 88–93.doi:10.1016/j.teln.2018.12.001

Prince Edward Island Occupational Therapy Society. (n.d.). *A history of the occupational therapy profession.* Charlottetown, PEI: Author.

Pringle, D., Green, L., & Johnson, S. (2004). *Nursing education in Canada: Historical review and current capacity.* Ottawa, ON: Nursing Sector Study Commission. Retrieved from https://www.nurseone.ca/~/media/nurseone/page-content/pdf-en/nursing_education_canada_e.pdf?la=en

Puplampu, K. P. (2004). The restructuring of higher education and part-time instructors: A theoretical and political analysis of undergraduate teaching in Canada. *Teaching in Higher Education, 9*(2), 171–182. doi:10.1080/1356251042000195376

Rajagopal, I. (2004). Tenuous ties: The limited-term full-time faculty in Canadian universities. *Review of Higher Education, 28*(1), 49–75.

Raymond, C., Profetto-McGrath, J., Myrick, F., & Strean, W. (2018). Balancing the seen and unseen: Nurse educator as role model for critical thinking. *Nurse Education in Practice, 4*(31), 41–47. doi:10.1016/j.nepr.2018.04.010

Ross-Gordon J. (2011). Research on adult learners: Supporting the needs of a student population that is no longer nontraditional. *Peer Review, 13*(1). Retrieved from https://www.aacu.org/publications-research/periodicals/research-adult-learners-supporting-needs-student-population-no

Semper, J., & Blasco, M. (2018). Revealing the hidden curriculum in higher education. *Studies in Philosophy and Education, 37*(3), 1–18. doi:10.1007/s11217-018-9608-5

Smith, C., Baldwin, C., & Schmidt, G. (2015). Student success centers: Leading the charge for change at community colleges. *Change: The Magazine of Higher Learning, 47*(2), 30–39. doi:10.1080/00091383.2015.1018087

Stone, R., Cooper, S., & Cant, R. (2013). The value of peer learning in undergraduate nursing education: A systematic review. *International Scholarly Research Notices,* Vol. 2013, Article ID 930901. doi:10.1155/2013/930901

Tyler, R. (1949). *Basic principles of curriculum and instruction.* Chicago, IL: University of Chicago Press.

Wraga, W. G. (2017). Understanding the Tyler rationale: *Basic principles of curriculum and instruction* in historical context. *Espacio, Tiempo y Educación, 4*(2), 227–252. doi:10.14516/ete.156

Wytenbroek, L., & Vandenberg, H. (2017). Reconsidering nursing's history during Canada 150. *Canadian Nurse, 133*(4), 120–124. Retrieved from https://www.canadian-nurse.com/en/articles/issues/2017/july-august-2017/reconsidering-nursings-history-during-canada-150

5

Maintaining Humanity in Technology-Rich Environments

Technology is just a tool. In terms of getting the kids working together and motivating them, the teacher is most important.

—Bill Gates in Bain & Zundans-Fraser, 2017, p. 137

In this chapter, we examine how educators can maintain humanity in the technology-rich learning environments that have become an essential part of life for most health professionals. How do we define such environments within a technology-rich world? As society has evolved over the decades, so have educational practices. Today we find a variety of classrooms, some that resemble the one-room schoolhouse of the 19th-century Western world, others that are fully virtual learning environments, and everything in between.

Of most interest in this chapter are the current face-to-face, blended, and online learning environments. Even if traditional face-to-face classrooms are not using digital technology for instruction, learners have their own technology at home and with them in the form of smartphones, laptops, and tablets. In most developed countries, postsecondary students have access to computers in classrooms, libraries, and computer labs, or they use their own equipment. The same is true for many practising health professionals. Technology is now ubiquitous in learning, and milieus are changing daily as educators introduce new technology-based learning activities and as computer scientists introduce new programs, apps, and technologies for learners to use. People are constantly adapting to new ways of communicating and learning.

Today parts or all aspects of a course, workshop, or orientation program can be offered online. As well, administrative activities in formal programs of higher education are frequently online, such as program applications, payments of fees, and transcripts for viewing. Learners have access to "frequently asked questions" electronically. Sometimes their questions are answered by a robot. Learners can choose from a plethora of online opportunities, including offerings such as massive open online courses (MOOCs). There are huge (and growing) repositories of books, journals, lessons, videos, podcasts, and so on available electronically to anyone anywhere without cost. Given the potential geographical, physical, and social distance that learners might experience when they utilize these advances in technology, how do educators develop and maintain relationships with learners in online learning environments?

Health-care service organizations and clinical agencies (which can include hospitals, public health units, and laboratories) are also learning environments for many health professionals. Health-care environments are usually rich in technology, with an abundance of pumps, machines, and monitors. The technologies that facilitate optimum patient/client care are changing constantly, with new devices and tools being adopted regularly. For example, the use of robots to provide patients/clients with companionship and support is a reality in some geriatric facilities, and other robots perform complex surgeries even though the surgeon is kilometres away from the patient.

"Technologies invite or afford specific patterns of thought, behaviour and valuing. They open up new possibilities for human action and foreclose or obscure others" (Vallor, 2018, p. 2). How can educators in the health professions maintain a human presence as they use online classrooms and clinical technologies to teach learners? How can educators choose wisely from among the multiple options available? How can we help learners to enhance real-world communications without becoming engulfed by the immediacy of social media? There are few if any straightforward answers to these vital questions. It is beyond the scope of this chapter to provide an in-depth explanation of all the technological supports available to educators to implement, particularly in online settings. Rather, we offer brief insights into approaches that educators can use to help make learning experiences with technology more humanized. We share suggestions drawn from our own practice as experienced online educators at Athabasca University, Canada's Open University. We note how social constructivist and humanist thinking can create a foundation for developing the human connections essential for meaningful learning. We offer strategies to humanize online learning environments. We include ideas that educators beginning to work with simulation activities might not have considered yet. We close the chapter with a snapshot of considerations that educators should heed when incorporating social media into their teaching approaches.

Social Constructivist and Humanist Thinking

In our practice as experienced online educators at Athabasca University, we are privileged to work extensively with learners in online classroom settings. In this section, we share insights from our "on the ground" work in technology-rich learning environments. In our view, social constructivist (SC) and humanist thinking provides a valuable theoretical foundation for establishing the human connections so necessary in technology-rich online learning environments.

Briefly, in social constructivism, knowledge is actively constructed (rather than acquired) through social interactions within a community of learners (Vygotsky, 1978). The social context of the learning environment is essential to learning success. Learning strategies focus on drawing from personal experiences and collaborations with others to achieve the assimilation of new information. Learners are motivated by goals that they set for themselves (intrinsic motivation) and by extrinsic motivation provided by the class community through expressions of support, encouragement, and praise for learning success. The educator's role is primarily that of facilitator, helping learners to work together to achieve their goals. Educators acknowledge that each person brings a unique perspective, experiences, and culture to the learning environment. As we have mentioned throughout the book, modelling appropriate and effective humanizing community-oriented behaviours is a task for SC-based educators.

Humanism focuses on human freedom, dignity, and individual potential and is a paradigm compatible with SC. According to humanism, people act intentionally and according to their personal values (Huitt, 2009). There is a focus on the whole experience and person rather than on segmented aspects, and the task for the person is to become self-actualized and autonomous

(Maslow, 2013). Teaching is student centered and personalized, and as in SC the educator is a facilitator who works to create a cooperative and supportive learning milieu that guides learners to achieve both affective domain and cognitive domain learning outcomes (Cooper, 1993).

Humanizing Online Learning Environments

Most postsecondary institutions now offer some online courses (or at least blended courses, with a portion of a course online and another part of it face to face). Some universities, such as Athabasca University, offer programs that are totally online, from admission application to graduation parchment. In such situations, learners are geographically isolated from one another and from their educators. There is a lack of physical presence, and participants can complete entire degree programs without ever sharing physical space with classmates or educators.

Online courses run the gamut from machine content broadcasts with no human instructor monitoring the class, to all-text presentations of content and discussion, to live video presentations with real-time discussion with all participants fully audio and video enabled. When selecting strategies to encourage human interaction with (and among) online students, the diversity in how online courses are offered needs to be considered. Self-paced courses not monitored by a human instructor do not elicit interaction (except when the student experiences a problem, and then there is contact for disciplinary, remedial, computer support, or other assistance between a student and an educator, administrator, or "help desk" staff member). This type of online course will require more effort by an educator to enhance the human element than an online class in which learners and educators regularly interact using audio and video. In the section that follows, we offer ideas for presenting introductory activities, facilitating interaction throughout courses, promoting teamwork, and offering feedback that can help educators to humanize online environments.

Introductions. The importance of introductions in teaching and learning interactions is often not given the time, effort, and attention required. Almost all successful human encounters begin with "hi, my name is. . . ." The other person reciprocates by sharing a greeting and his or her name. This basic human nicety is important in facilitating dialogue and discussion and learning. If we do not know the other person's name, how do we ask that person a question in a respectful way? How do you recognize whom you are addressing if you do not know that person's name? People enjoy hearing their names; they are symbols of who they are, among the most personal things about them, and many take pride in their names. Taking the time to get to know the names of other people in a class is an essential foundation for important learning experiences that will occur later in the course.

Spending time on introductions is congruent with SC and humanist theoretical foundations of learning. If the social context is where most learning occurs (a pillar of SC), then participants need to know one another on social and personal levels. This is a precursor to collaborative learning that will occur throughout the course. Likewise, humanists believe that a cooperative and supportive learning milieu is conducive to achieving affective domain and cognitive domain learning outcomes. For class members to be supportive of one another, and for educators to know learners personally so that they can provide individualized support, meaningful and memorable introductions seem to be essential.

With the use of technology, it is now relatively easy in asynchronous online classes for the educator and learners to introduce themselves to one another using video. There are many options, from YouTube to Zoom to other platforms. In synchronous learning environments, a group session on Zoom, Adobe Connect, Skype, or other similar programs will afford a chance for participants to meet one another, and these interactions can be the beginnings of relationships that develop further throughout the class.

If real-time video is not available for introductions, tools such as Swoop will allow participants to create and post polished static presentations with words and pictures. Using these strategies, introductions can be meaningful for the participants. The lack of opportunity for real-time interaction is a disadvantage of this approach. However, since photos are a part of these "presentations," these introductions can be more meaningful than a post in a course forum or an email introduction.

Introductions are not interactions until someone responds. The tone for the course will be set by the way in which educators introduce themselves and respond to learners' introductions. An educator can convey enthusiasm for the course content (and a passion for teaching) with a positive, upbeat, and perhaps even humorous introduction. By asking learners individualized questions based on their introductions, educators display a concern for each person and a genuine interest in learners as people first. Below is one technique that educators can use to enhance the humanizing potential of introductions.

Facilitation. Following thoughtful introductions, educators facilitate and support interaction throughout a course. Originally, Athabasca University provided distance instruction in a way that mirrored correspondence courses. Interactions with learners were primarily via written comments on mailed assignments and during weekly office hours when individual learners could telephone educators (named tutors at our institution) to ask them questions. Learners could sense the humanity of their tutors through their encouraging words on assignments and through rare telephone conversations.

From this correspondence course model, the university moved to online courses (synchronous and asynchronous) in which learners primarily read course materials and answered discussion questions by posting written comments in online forms. Other learners and tutors could respond to learners' posts with additional written comments and questions.

At Athabasca University, there were often discussions among online faculty about how much to participate in these online class discussions. It is a real art to make your presence known, encourage the students, and not hinder their discussion. We have found that, instead of tutors adding content that learners are missing (thereby cutting off the opportunity for them to do so), participants find greater learning opportunities when tutors offer gentle encouragement, ask thoughtful questions that extend the discussion, and provide praise for critical thinking. Many tutors provide regular summaries (written or video) of recent class discussions, giving them the opportunity to highlight important points and allowing them to introduce concepts that might have been missed. Sometimes these weekly summaries lead to an overview of the next topic of discussion. Any learner-specific critique or encouragement is provided via private communication, usually via course mail or regular mail.

The correspondence courses had live phone office hours, and online courses can accommodate that. Individual or group sessions with the tutor can be verbal or audio/video with the technology commonly available now. As well, with most of the online communication software, the interactions can be recorded for future reference or for learners unable to attend a session in real time.

SC and humanist theories are congruent with these approaches to teaching in online courses. For example, SC purports that learning is an active rather than a passive process. As learners engage in online discussions (either synchronously or asynchronously), they actively engage with the course content. When course participants (tutors and learners) comment on one another's posts or ask each other questions to further the discussion, this is active learning and collaboration, both hallmarks of SC. The opportunities afforded to tutors to react to, question, and praise each learner's contributions through email are congruent with a humanist theory of learning. Learners feel respected and supported when educators take the time to provide this individualized feedback. Try the following strategy to enact this humanizing approach.

A STRATEGY TO TRY

"Today I Noticed" Emails

To humanize the online classroom, educators can make a deliberate effort to observe and comment on something positive about each learner each week. These positive observations can be delivered through personalized course mail. It is helpful to keep a chart showing learners' names and the weeks that the course or workshop is offered. Each time the educator sends a learner a "today I noticed" email, it can be checked off on the chart. This way all learners receive recognition on a regular basis. The email can be as short as one or two sentences,

> but the message needs to include specific observations and details, be genuine in tone, be positive, and be signed by the educator.

Teamwork. This is a foundational element of humanist online learning environments. We all know that both educators and learners have a love/hate relationship with group assignments. As tutors at Athabasca University who embrace SC and humanist educational theory, we want to encourage the teamwork and collaboration that undergird group projects. New technologies make the experience of group work easier, more accessible, and potentially a better learning experience. Learners can work simultaneously or asynchronously on a single document or presentation. They can meet online in asynchronous or real-time discussions, and they can engage in collaborative writing or work on their own sections of a group assignment.

We also know that online group projects come with the potential for interpersonal issues. However, within the framework of SC, providing opportunities for learners to collaborate is fundamental to learning. When a group project has the potential to affect each learner's final grade, the stakes are high, and tolerance for non-contributing (or weak) group members can be limited. It is important that the educator provides clear expectations and guidelines for the group project to optimize students' experience.

For example, how groups are formed can set them up for success or result in angst and detract from the potential positive outcomes of collaborative work. The educator needs to answer the following questions. Should learners choose their own groups, or should the educator assign groups? If the educator creates groups, should members be assigned randomly or strategically? For example, should all learners in the same time zone be grouped together? An educator who seeks to create a positive environment for online learners to engage in group work faces many choices.

One suggestion that educators can follow when forming groups is to assign participants into groups as they log in to a course. For example, for groups of four, the first four students who log in to the course once it opens become a group. This strategy creates groups with similar patterns of participation and possibly levels of motivation. Some would argue that this approach is not fair because most of the "keen" learners are in the first group formed, whereas the less active (and perhaps less engaged) learners form a subsequent group. However, from our observations at Athabasca University, when learners share similar patterns of participation (as evident from when they log in to a course), motivation, enthusiasm, and drive, this approach to group membership can promote a sense of enjoyment and satisfaction among them. Are you interested in a creative way to form groups for this experience? Consider the following idea.

A STRATEGY TO TRY

Ideas for Forming Groups

To humanize the online classroom, in part by respecting the dignity and individuality of each student, online instructors must become skilled at group formation. Group work is valued for the opportunities that it provides for active learning, collaboration, and learning in a social context. Groups can be formed using the following strategies: by birth month (e.g., January to June, July to December), by region (e.g., western Canada, eastern Canada, the Maritimes), by discipline (e.g., nurses), or by preference (e.g., cat lovers, dog lovers). All of these strategies are random. Strategic groups can be formed using the following approaches: according to current GPA (e.g., higher GPA, lower GPA), number of courses completed (e.g., four or more courses completed, fewer than four courses completed), time of first login (e.g., students assigned to groups in the order in which they first log in to the new course), or group topic preferences (e.g., the instructor provides topics for group work, and students sign up for the topic that interests them most).

Feedback. An important aspect of educator-learner relationships in any educational experience is feedback. In settings of higher education, such as our university, we strive to provide feedback to learners in ways that will strengthen our relationships with them. We know that learners respond positively to specific and detailed feedback on their assignments (Balaji & Chakrabarti, 2010). Can you imagine spending all that time writing a paper or preparing a presentation and receiving nothing more than a grade and a "well done" comment? What if you receive a mark well below what you expected and the instructor has not provided any justification for the mark (or any ideas for improvement)? When this occurs in online classes, the lack of personal contact makes the scenario even more troublesome for students. They might experience an array of dehumanizing emotions.

In part, the potential in online courses for the feedback experience to be negative is because students submit (and receive feedback on) assignments electronically. This eliminates educator-learner face-to-face interaction (e.g., questions asked and additional comments made), which can be an important part of the assessment and learning processes in traditional courses. For online learners, course technology automates the process of assignment submission and return. However, the software usually offers an opportunity for learners and educators to add personal comments to the assignment documents. These more informal and personalized aspects of the assessment process should be used to help humanize assessment. Assessment and feedback can be made even more individualized if educators provide audio feedback on each learner's assignment. Audio comments can be embedded directly into the document that a learner submits. Most online learners appreciate this type of response and acknowledge that hearing the tone of the educator's voice can help them to understand the intent of evaluative messages. Furthermore, audio feedback is often more complete since it takes the educator less time to say a comment than to type a comment. Audio comments feel more personalized since "voice is particularly impactful in our text-based world" (Morrison, April 6, 2013, para. 1).

Another voice-based type of feedback used by online educators is an audio (or video) comment addressed to an entire class explaining the grading of an assignment. In this process, the educator can explain decisions about certain aspects of the assessment, describe the class average, and review weaknesses and strengths common to most (or all) of the papers. Although the audio/video group message is not as personalized as an individualized recording, it still relays a feeling to the group that there is a real educator out there who received and reviewed their assignments. An approach to providing audio feedback is described below.

Speak to Learners

To individualize feedback on written assignments, try embedding audio or video files when returning documents to learners. Using audio comments (instead of or in addition to text-based comments) saves time and allows learners to hear their educator's voice (tone, cadence, accent) and know that there is a real person who has graded their work. There are many tools available for providing this personalized audio feedback. Choose one that is easy to use and share with learners. Experiment with using the voice recorder app on your smartphone or other free apps such as Evernote.

Simulation

Simulation is interactive technology. There are many types of simulation that range from low to high technology (depending on the complexity of the equipment). In programs for educating health professionals, the main type of simulation used is high-tech human patient simulators. Educators believe that such simulators provide opportunities for authentic clinical practice experiences without the risk of endangering a live patient/client.

As far back as 2001, academics were enthusiastic about patient simulators, though research was limited. One of the first simulators used to complete a cardiopulmonary resuscitation course was the manikin Rescue Annie, on which learners practised compressions. Today's simulators are much more sophisticated and allow learners to practise on virtual manikins of all types while online (or face to face). Learners report that these simulation experiences are beneficial, saying that they are powerful learning opportunities that "increase ethical decision-making, confidence, and effective advocacy while also building courage to overcome fears and defend ethical practice" (Krautscheid, 2017, p. 55).

The technology that simulation introduces into the learning environment (online and face to face) has become an essential and permanent aspect of health-care education. No doubt simulation will become even more essential as a teaching and learning tool as technology advances. Furthering the technology of simulation is the lack of physical clinical placement learning options for learners. Traditionally, pre-service learners spent parts of their programs in hospitals and other clinical agencies where they practised skills on real people (usually under the watchful eye of a graduated professional). Now such traditional learning opportunities are becoming rare, and the number of learners is increasing, meaning that as simulation becomes increasingly realistic and accessible learners are spending more of their practice time with simulated patients/clients.

Simulation learning is often immersive, and it provides a way for learners to obtain real-time feedback on their actions as the manikin reacts to their movements. Simulation evokes and replicates many aspects of the real world in a fully interactive fashion. Patient/client manikins speak, cry out in pain, ask questions, respond to questions and actions by the caregiver, vomit, bleed, and even give birth.

Skilled educators need to be cognizant of using simulation technology in ways that allow learners to feel human emotions such as empathy. In other words, educators can take steps to make what is essentially a piece of plastic as authentically human as possible in the minds and hearts of learners. Strategies such as choosing realistic scenarios, personalizing the manikin or model (providing a name, demographic details, etc.), encouraging collaboration with other health-care team members, and expecting mistakes (this is real life) can make the scenarios realistic human experiences. Scenarios can also be altered to challenge the specific learning needs and goals of a particular learner to help personalize the experience. Giving the manikin a personal history rather than simply a medical condition helps learners to focus on affective domain learning outcomes as well as on cognitive and psychomotor knowledge.

It is important to emphasize that learners are continually observing how educators behave in relation to simulation. Educators are role models and have an important part to play in making the scenarios realistic and the most effective learning experience possible. Having clear roles for each person who participates in a simulation is important for learning and making sure that the scenario is realistic and that everyone has a chance to participate in it fully and immersively.

Learner anxiety. Although many educators talk about the decreased risk to a live patient/client that simulation learning provides, few mention that participating in simulation experiences can bring risks for learners. Some learners report extreme anxiety when they are asked to perform in a simulated scenario. Where does humane interaction fit into this picture? If we are humane educators, then we must anticipate that some learners will experience more anxiety than others (some to the point that they will freeze and be unable to react). Learners, after all, are asked to be actors. Simulations are usually completed in front of peers and educators, and they are often recorded (videotaped) for playback (for either formative or summative assessment). Anxiety is accentuated when learners are asked to suspend reality and behave as though the manikin is a real person. They must make decisions, act, communicate, and evaluate situations while "on stage." In an integrated review of ten research articles on anxiety and performance in a simulated setting, Al-Ghareeb, Cooper, and McLennan (2017) concluded that simulation can be a profound stressor for learners, that the anxiety can interfere with the stated benefits of simulation, and that simulation practice can actually create a negative non-learning experience for learners.

So we have studies of learners who claim that simulation exercises help them to build confidence and others who have extreme difficulty with anxiety when performing such exercises and need confidence building. Performing successfully in a simulation is the highest level of Bloom's taxonomy, fitting his descriptor "characterization" well. One of his characterizations is knowing how to seek needed help (Bloom & Krathwohl, 1956). Educators who use simulation (either online or face to face) need to be aware that for some learners the anxiety of being a participant in a simulation experience can be an enhancer, whereas for others the anxiety detracts from learning and can have negative consequences for the learner outside the learning experience. Educators need to have an array of strategies to help prevent the negative effects of anxiety in simulation learning.

As a beginning, all of the strategies in this book that encourage learner self-valuing, help to decrease learner isolation, and promote learner-educator and learner-learner interaction can be helpful in ensuring success in simulation exercises, but additional strategies are needed. For example, it is common practice to have prebriefing and debriefing exercises as part of simulation experiences.

Dr. Nicole Harder, an assistant professor in the College of Nursing at the Rady Faculty of Health Sciences at the University of Manitoba, is the faculty member in charge of the Nursing Simulation Lab. Besides her research in the field of simulation, Harder is the editor-in-chief of the journal *Clinical*

Simulation in Nursing. According to her (N. Harder, personal communication, September 17, 2018), learner anxiety can also stem from the specific simulation. The simulations that most frequently trigger emotions in learners are dying scenarios and those dealing with suicide. Harder structures the pre- and post-briefing conferences in her lab around psychological safety in relation to these especially stressful simulations. The strategy described below outlines safe words for use in simulation scenarios.

A STRATEGY TO TRY

Safe Words and Activities in Simulation Scenarios

A strategy that can humanize the experience for learners in simulation experiences is to provide a "safe word" for them to say if they need to remove themselves from a simulation. Other activities include allowing learners to choose being an observer rather than an actor until their confidence increases; having a counsellor on site to support students who experience anxiety; helping learners to find and discuss personal coping strategies; helping students to talk about their anxiety levels; keeping learners in the same small group throughout the simulation experience so that they develop comfort with and support from each other; encouraging students to push themselves by making simulation free from evaluation; helping learners to understand that mistakes are expected when problem solving in an unknown situation; stopping simulation for mini-debriefing right after something significant happens; and consciously pairing anxious learners with peers who are less anxious (but supportive).

Reflection. This is a critical aspect of any successful learning experience and should not be overlooked in simulation activities. Educators need to be able to identify learners who might be at risk of simulation-induced anxiety. By knowing learners well in advance of simulation activities, educators can have some idea of who might need additional help in those activities. Unfortunately, many educational groups who participate in simulation activities are large, and learners move from educator to educator for different courses and workshops. Keeping class groups small and having the same cohort of learners with the same educator for all simulations during a term can be helpful. Dr. Harder has a large group of learners who go through the Sim Lab every term, and she says that by the end of their six-week lab experience she knows them all. Harder states that it is important that a reflective activity be implemented prior to simulation to identify learner anxiety levels so that any potential dehumanizing effects can be prevented. The strategy below describes a reflective exercise that could be adapted to many teaching situations.

A STRATEGY TO TRY

"Imagine if. . . ."

Before learners engage in simulation activities, have them engage in a reflective writing exercise. Describe a simulation experience by including all of the details of the "patient," reactions, outcomes, et cetera. Alternatively, show learners a video of a former group of learners completing a simulation exercise (perhaps a group from a previous year). Make sure that you have appropriate permissions to use such an example for teaching purposes. After showing the video or describing the scenario and experience, have learners "imagine if . . . you were the learner in the video/scenario." Ask them to reflect on how they would feel, how they would respond, what they would be thinking about, and have them write these feelings/thoughts down. Facilitate a group discussion and sharing of reflections.

Anxiety reduction. Educators in the health professions are usually aware of how anxiety can affect learning, particularly in clinical contexts. Techniques that educators have found valuable in reducing their own anxieties and those of their learners in other situations can be implemented during simulation activities. Any technique that acknowledges how anxiety can be a positive influence on learning rather than a distraction can help.

Additionally, we suggest three that might be of interest. First, consider exploring autogenic training, a form of deep relaxation that has been successfully tested as an anxiety-reducing technique prior to simulation exercises (Holland, Gosselin, & Malcahy, 2017). Second, at institutions with counselling services, invite a counsellor to speak to learners before simulations begin. The presence of a counsellor and knowing that services are available normalize the process of seeking help if and when it is needed. For learners, understanding their own feelings and knowing that they are not alone in their responses allow learner-to-learner support to develop as well. Third, as educators we are aware that learners can experience simulation-induced anxiety for several reasons. We can prepare the students for that possibility, and we can watch for evidence of an issue. We are prepared to act.

Despite the anxiety-inducing potential of simulation activities, they can be powerful tools to help learners understand how to be humane with each other, with the manikin, and with other actors in the simulation. For example, simulations can be specifically designed to elicit feelings of empathy and expressions of compassion in learners. These affective domain learning outcomes are often very challenging to "teach," and a simulation in which the educator makes the scenario real can be an avenue for teaching and learning these often nebulous but essential health-care competencies.

SOCIAL MEDIA

Social media applications are everywhere now, including in courses and work-shops for health professionals offered by institutions of higher education and clinical agencies. Of course, even email is a type of social media. Few educators are not involved with internet-based communication with their learners, either individually or as a group. As well, educators in the health professions must teach and encourage digital literacy. Learners (online and face to face) engage in web searches to complete assignments and prepare for simulations and practice experiences, and many postsecondary institutions have online libraries. In progressive settings, learners are now being required to create websites about themselves and their course work (e-portfolios), communicate via Twitter and/or Facebook within their courses, and collate information on sites such as Pinterest and share it with others. Course work is also being shared via podcasts and blogs to help make assessment authentic.

Professionalism. In online settings in which health professionals are educated, addressing professionalism in social media is a key consideration. Educators have many social media applications and search engines available to augment their teaching and learning. How can we as educators help learners to use these technologies (both the advantages and the disadvantages), teach them professionalism while interacting virtually, remind them of the ethics of using social media, and ensure that they use these tools optimally to enhance both patient/client care and their own lifelong learning? In the strategy below, we suggest an icebreaker that educators can implement with learners in pre-service and in-service programs. A key goal of the activity is to initiate discussions of professionalism in online environments. All learners (and educators) should be aware of their digital footprints. The strategy below outlines an activity that all can use to review their digital footprints regularly.

A STRATEGY TO TRY

Check Your Digital Footprint

In the early stages of an educational experience, as participants are beginning their work together, ask them to choose several search engines and search their names in each of them. Invite them to compile a list of what they found "out there" about them that surprised or worried them. Ask them to do some research on how to protect their digital footprints and to share the strategies that they discover with others in the learning group.

Understanding policies. Most postsecondary institutions and clinical agencies have (or are developing) policies related to social media. As new practices using social media are integrated into educational experiences for health professionals, the opportunities and disadvantages are not well researched. We assume that there are benefits in sharing our work with our peers and in some cases on the World Wide Web. We also know that there are issues related to the overuse of technology, especially the potential negative effects on interpersonal relationships. As educators, it is important that we consider the impacts of social media on our teaching approaches and classrooms.

The technologies (Facebook, Pinterest, Twitter, etc.) are tools and can be used in many ways. What we are interested in is how they affect human interactions in educational scenarios. In their discussion, Schmitt, Sims-Giddens, and Booth (2012) lead us to think about several actions in which educators can engage to smooth the learning process for their students. Most important is for educators, and the organizations that they work in, to have a social media policy. The development of such a policy facilitates discussion on the appropriate use of these technologies and the issues related to them. In the strategy that follows, we call on educators to increase their own awareness as well as that of their learners regarding social media policies at their organizations.

A STRATEGY TO TRY

Treasure Hunt: Find Your Social Media Policy

Ask learners in the course or workshop that you facilitate to find the social media policy of their professional association and/or the educational institution or clinical agency in which they work and/or learn. If they are affiliated with multiple organizations, then they can find several policies and compare them in a written assignment (blog post or essay) or share key points of the policy or policies as part of a group discussion.

Introduce technologies individually. New technologies can seem overwhelming to educators and learners alike. Schmitt et al. (2012) suggest that new technologies should be introduced one at a time in the educational milieu. Doing so gives educators time to know their learners well before using these strategies in teaching and learning. If all learners (and educators) are tech savvy, then perhaps this initial assessment period is not as important. However, in some organizations, the average age of learners is higher, and many have not been embedded in social media technology for long. The gradual introduction of social media use in course and workshop classrooms also gives learners time to grow into the practices required. If learners are familiar with the technologies before they are used in activities or assignments, then they can focus on presenting their ideas (and learning) as opposed to fretting about using (or learning to use) the actual technology.

Privacy settings. Finally, and importantly, learners should be provided with privacy settings for any required technology used for educational purposes in courses or workshops. Some activities (e.g., following a health professional on Twitter) require access to the web. Learners must be aware of where their comments and posts can be seen. They might be very reluctant to have their names and information available to anyone who wants to find them, and frequently there are legitimate reasons for this concern. Other learners think that it is important to share their academic work as much as possible as a contribution to public good. Caution should always guide an educator who chooses to ask learners to use social media in educational activities or to share their learning with the educator, other learners, or the world.

CONCLUSION

Technology has changed the world of learners and educators. Social constructivist and humanist thinking can help educators to navigate this brave new world. Educators who use technology need to keep the pillars of SC thinking (learning occurs in active, collaborative, and socially rich environments) and the tenets of humanist thinking (learners need to be supported and treated with dignity, learning should be individualized, and affective learning is essential) in mind.

Technology in its various forms (including online learning environments, simulation activities, and social media) can enhance learning in many ways, but it also brings with it the potential to tarnish the vital human element essential to education in the health professions. In this chapter, we discussed ways in which educators can underscore that vital human element. Based on our experience in educating university students in online classrooms at Athabasca University, we encourage our fellow educators to create human connections during course or workshop introduction activities, to consistently facilitate and support interaction, to integrate teamwork, and to provide personalized feedback that includes suggestions for improvement.

Extensive literature exists to guide educators through the simulation activities that they implement with learners. We suggest that recognizing learners' anxiety, encouraging reflection, and providing opportunities for learners to participate in anxiety reduction activities during both pre-briefing and post-briefing of simulation sessions are especially helpful. When educators integrate social media into technology-rich learning environments, we recommend that they pay special attention to issues of professionalism, organizational policies, sequencing, and privacy.

We can no longer pretend that educators and learners can thrive without knowledge of and practice with educational technologies. In the futuristic work of Harari (2018), readers are invited to imagine a technology-infused, science fiction–like world. Such a world might be imminent, and it is useful to heed his advice to educators. Harari writes that "most important of all will be the ability to deal with change, learn new things and preserve your mental balance in unfamiliar situations" (p. 266).

REFERENCES

Al-Ghareeb, A., Cooper, S., & McLennan, L. (2017). Anxiety and clinical performance in simulated settings in undergraduate health professionals' education: An integrated review. *Clinical Simulation in Learning, 13*(10), 478–491. doi:10.1016/j.ecns.2017.05.015

Bain, A., & Zundans-Fraser, L. (2017). *The self-organizing university: Designing the higher education organization for quality learning and teaching.* Singapore: Springer. doi:10.1007/978-981-10-4917-0

Balaji, M. S., & Chakrabarti, D. (2010). Student interactions in online discussion forum: Empirical research from "media richness theory" perspective. *Journal of Interactive Online Learning, 9*(1), 1–22. Retrieved from https://pdfs. semanticscholar.org/a7c1/5dfdba9eff739a38dfdd6eed83d380280f98.pdf

Bloom, B. S., & Krathwohl, D. R. (1956). *Taxonomy of educational objectives: The classification of educational goals, by a committee of college and university examiners. Handbook I: Cognitive domain.* New York, NY: Longmans, Green.

Cooper, P. A. (1993). Paradigm shifts in designed instruction: From behaviourism to cognitivism to constructivism. *Educational Technology, 33*(5), 12–19.

Harari, Y. (2018). *21 Lessons for the 21st Century.* New York, NY: Spiegel & Grau.

Holland, B., Gosselin, K., & Malcahy, A. (2017). The effect of autogenic training on self-efficacy, anxiety, and performance on nursing student simulation. *Nursing Education Perspectives, 38*(2), 87–89. doi:10.1097/01.NEP.0000000000000110

Huitt, W. (2009). Humanism and open education. *Educational Psychology Interactive.* Valdosta, GA: Valdosta State University. Retrieved from http://www. edpsycinteractive.org/topics/affect/humed.html

Krautscheid, L. (2017). Embedding microethical dilemmas in high-fidelity simulation scenarios. *Journal of Nursing Education, 56*(1), 55–58. doi:10.3928/01484834-20161219-11

Maslow, A. H. (2013). *Toward a psychology of being.* New York, NY: Start Publishing.

Morrison, D. (April 6, 2013). 'Speaking to students' with audio feedback in online courses. *Online Learning Insights* [Blog]. Retrieved from https:// onlinelearninginsights.wordpress.com/2013/04/06/speaking-to-students-with-audio-feedback-in-online-courses/

Schmitt, T., Sims-Giddens, S., & Booth, R. (2012). Social media use in nursing education. *The Online Journal of Nursing Issues, 17*(3). Retrieved from https:// www.ncbi.nlm.nih.gov/pubmed/23036058

Vallor, S. (2018). *Technology and the virtues: A philosophical guide to a future worth wanting*. New York, NY: Oxford University Press.

Vygotsky, L. (1978). *Mind in society*. Cambridge, MA: Harvard University Press.

6

Maintaining Motivation in Teaching

*Robots are not people. They are mechanically more perfect than
we are, they have astonishing intellectual capacity, but they have
no soul.*

—Karel Čapek, 1926, p. 7–8

In this final chapter, we explore an issue that many educators grapple with but
might not acknowledge or feel comfortable addressing: that is, maintaining
motivation. Excellent educators are expected to be enthusiastic, committed to
learners' success, and motivated to keep their classes or workshops lively. Yet
even excellent educators can find their motivation waning at times. Increasing numbers of learners, seemingly chaotic clinical learning environments,
and mounting workplace expectations can all affect motivation. As a result,
educators who are truly excellent can also slip into an emotional state more
robotic than human and thus less humane. In fact, an ebb and flow in motivation is common in life. In our view, when people experience low motivation,
it is simply another reflection of being human. Bringing excitement back and
beginning to resolve issues related to motivation are an opportunity to grow
and develop in innovative ways.

Moving beyond feelings of low motivation is not easy. As a tentative
starting point in not becoming a robot, consider these questions. Do you
think that your teaching approach has not changed since you started teaching
several years ago? Do you look forward to a new course or workshop with

enthusiasm, or are you more likely to turn to a new group of learners with a sense of ho-hum? Do you ever feel like a robot just doing what is needed to get through a learning experience? If you are becoming a sleepwalking, unenthusiastic educator, then this chapter might be timely. Perhaps you are losing your motivation to excel at your career, or, worse, you are experiencing a syndrome such as burnout or rust-out.

Educator burnout and rust-out have become topics in the education literature. An early definition of burnout put forward by Edelwich and Brodsky is "a continuously increasing loss in idealism, energy and purpose" in one's work (1980, p. 6). Maslach, Schaufeli, and Leiter (2001) added the idea of emotional exhaustion and depersonalization to the definition of burnout, and Shirom (1989) emphasized the negative emotional reaction that happens in someone experiencing burnout. The outcomes associated with burnout include physical, social, emotional, and psychological challenges that can have negative effects on people's personal and professional well-being.

Burnout has been studied in many populations but is most often associated with caring professions such as health care, education, and human service careers in which practitioners have close relationships with other people and high levels of work stress. Bridgeman, Bridgeman, and Barone (2018) note that burnout is composed of physical and behavioural symptoms (e.g., anger, frustration, suspicion) that compound over time and influence one's career ambitions in a negative way. Burnout is said to result from factors such as excessive workload, perception of unfair rewards, lack of a sense of control over work, and incongruence between organizational and personal values (Bridgeman et al., 2018; Dall'Ora, Reinius, & Griffiths, 2020).

"Rust-out" is a less commonly used term but equally negative for practitioners and learners taught by someone experiencing this condition. Leider and Buchholz (1995, p. 7) introduced the rust-out syndrome and defined it as a "slow process of deterioration of motivation through the disuse of an individual's potentials." In some ways, rust-out is the opposite of burnout, with burnout caused by overdoing and rust-out attributed to being under-challenged or bored. Clouston (2015) describes rust-out as the boredom-based counterpart of burnout since it occurs when workers are no longer challenged in positive ways by their work and consequently become uninterested in and apathetic about doing their jobs well. This boredom can be stressful and lead to psychological and physical symptoms (Brown, 2015). If the emotional difficulties created by rust-out are not dealt with, then the outcome is stagnation and loss of a sense of purpose in the individual. Poor-quality work is usually the consequence, to the detriment of the education provided to learners.

Both burnout and rust-out, if left unchecked, have negative influences on job satisfaction. Being satisfied with one's career is an important precursor to quality curricula delivery and influences recruitment and retention of educators (Cowin & Moroney, 2018). In other words, when educators experience their work as personally fulfilling, they are more successful in their careers and more likely to remain in their current positions. Satisfied educators find meaning in their work and feel compelled to continue to do it in an exemplary way. Riley (2018) concluded that there is a relationship between overall wellness (in part, freedom from syndromes such as burnout and rust-out) and job satisfaction. Additionally, learners benefit when educators are satisfied in their roles.

How can pre-service and in-service educators in the health professions prevent rust-out and burnout and achieve job satisfaction? Some educators seem to become more passionate, engaged, and skilled over time. Perhaps the secret is the successful creation and maintenance of human connections. That is, the educators who get the sense (or other indications) that they have real connections with learners in their classes might be on the way to achieving at least a certain level of career fulfillment, thereby minimizing the possibility of the negative sequalae.

There is limited research available on the importance of educator job satisfaction and engagement and the potential influence that they have on the quality of the learning milieu and on educators' well-being (Milburn-Shaw & Walker, 2017). We believe that, when educators do feel satisfied, motivated, and engaged, they can create an environment in which learners thrive. In this chapter, we comment on how the community of inquiry model discussed in Chapter 3 can provide insights into maintaining motivation in educational settings. We emphasize how engagement can make the difference between an excellent educator and a robotic teacher. We explain how human connections that count include attending to the "little things," affirming the value of others, and sharing humour appropriately.

It can be difficult to understand what motivation means to educators and how they can best remain motivated and not become robotic teachers. As a way of gaining insight into what motivation can look like for educators, we begin with a story shared by an academic who teaches health profession students online. She had been teaching students for years, mostly face to face but more recently online. At first, she thought that it would be challenging to form bonds with learners and really get to know them as she had in traditional classes. This experienced educator changed her perception. One day she received an email from a student in her group:

> I just want to thank you for helping me through this semester. I didn't tell you, but I have been going through a really tough time. I had my second miscarriage about two weeks into the term. We have been going through treatments and trying to conceive for several years. This loss was a real blow to our hope for a family. Then we were victims of the flooding, [and] having to leave our house and possessions and spend time in the evacuation centre was scary and disheartening. Finally, as we got back home and resettled (thankfully our house was not damaged), my mom was diagnosed with ALS. The turmoil I have experienced this term has been unmatched by anything I have experienced before.
>
> At times I thought of dropping the course, perhaps even dropping out of the program, but I kept going. Why—because of you. I am not sure how you knew I needed words of encouragement and flexibility with assignment dates, but you must have a sense of the stress your students are experiencing. Your frequent reassuring emails, seemingly written just to me, made me feel that you cared about my learning and about me as a fellow human being. Your abundant thoughtful comments on my assignments both taught me important content and motivated me to try harder to do well. The challenging and engaging learning activities you shared piqued my interest and encouraged me to make time for my course during all the trauma in my life. Thank you—you really made a difference for me.

This story gives us hints about the ways that educators maintain their motivation to do their job in an exemplary way. This chapter is about how you, as an educator of health professionals, can remain motivated to provide excellent teaching and keep from becoming a burned-out or rusted-out robotic educator. About how you can remain energized and inspired by your work.

About how you can continue to provide excellent learner-focused teaching when there seems to be a din of negativity, the challenge of constant change, and seemingly relentless competing urgencies threatening your plans and best intentions. About how you can keep from becoming a robotic teacher, an educator who follows directions and scripts and curricula but is absent in heart, an educator who succumbs to the syndromes of rust-out and burnout.

Insights from the CoI model. Garrison, Anderson, and Archer (2000) developed the community of inquiry model. In Chapter 3, we explained how the model provides educators with important insights as they create and enhance relationships between educators and learners. The model also provides insight into how educators can maintain their motivation to remain excellent at what they do. To review, the CoI model posits that "a community of inquiry is a group of individuals who collaboratively engage in purposeful critical discourse and reflection to construct personal meaning and confirm mutual understanding" (Garrison et al., p. 1). There are three elements in the model: social presence, teaching presence, and cognitive presence. In brief, social presence is the ability of educators and learners to create relationships and to share their personalities in the learning environment. Teaching presence is the way in which educators structure and facilitate learning experiences to create meaningful learning. And cognitive presence is the aspect of an educational milieu in which learners engage in individual reflection and shared discourse (Garrison et al.).

When educators successfully create learning experiences in which there are social presence, teaching presence, and cognitive presence, they are likely to feel satisfied that they have done their job well. Learners in such a situation experience meaningful learning and develop interpersonal relationships with other learners and with the educator that they value. The creation of a healthy CoI can fuel the cycle of career satisfaction and positive student outcomes foundational to preventing and remedying educator burnout and rust-out.

Robotic teachers are not likely to attain a high level of social presence, especially when they guard against sharing their personalities with learners (however inadvertently). In turn, learners who do not get the sense that there is a "real" educator guiding their learning can also be reluctant to open up and create relationships in the learning milieu. The result can be a deficit in achieving the social presence element of the CoI.

Likewise, teaching presence (and the design and creation of meaningful learning experiences) are not usual outcomes if the educator is bored or uninspired. It takes energy, optimism, and enthusiasm for an educator to establish teaching presence. Rusted-out and burned-out individuals have a serious deficit in these areas. The omission of teaching presence means that yet another element of the CoI can be lacking in such situations.

Finally, cognitive presence, or the establishment of opportunities for learners to engage in sustained reflection and discourse, is in many ways dependent on the creation of teaching presence and social presence in the classroom. When elements of the CoI are minimal or non-existent, it becomes challenging for learners to fully engage in meaningful learning.

Perhaps if educators can make strong connections with learners through social presence, and perceive that they are engaging in high-quality teaching by attending to the elements of teaching presence, then learners will be guided and supported to engage in sustained reflection and meaningful discourse (cognitive presence). As we will highlight later in this chapter, seemingly the small actions and strategies that skilled educators use often become the catalysts for these positive outcomes and the establishment of a healthy CoI. Self-awareness is an essential first step. The strategy below outlines a beginning step for educators.

A STRATEGY TO TRY

Checking Your Rust!

Self-awareness is essential in recognizing and reversing rust-out. Set a date (perhaps the first day of each semester or orientation program) to have a serious sit-down talk with yourself and look for signs of rust-out. Choose a comfortable, quiet setting where you can have some valued thinking time. Ask yourself questions such as am I truly present (socially, teaching, and cognitively) with my learners? Am I keen to try new things? Do I feel good about what I have accomplished at the end of each workday? Do I still feel a spark of excitement when I start a new learning experience?

If the answers to these questions leave you feeling that you might be experiencing rust-out, then make a plan to address these situations. It starts with an honest assessment of your teaching paradigm. Reflecting on insights offered by the CoI model might be the trigger that you need to scrape off the rust.

Educator engagement and the effect on learners. Educators are the keystone of the educational process and have a direct impact on learners and their learning experiences (Alpaslan, Bozgeyikli, & Avci, 2017). Most fully engaged educators love their job, work willingly, establish healthy relationships with their learners, and conduct the educational process successfully (Karahan, 2018). When educators achieve these outcomes and are satisfied with their careers and work performance, learners benefit in several ways. For example, learners who learn from engaged educators are more successful in achieving learning outcomes, gaining on measures of emotional intelligence over a term, and developing critical thinking skills (Alvandi, Mehrdad, & Karimi, 2015). On the reverse side, disengaged educators (demonstrated by indolence and offensiveness) cause learners' interest and engagement to wane (Broeckelman-Post et al., 2016). Educator behaviour (or misbehaviour) influences student behaviour and how students experience the learning environment.

Educator engagement and the effect on teachers. Educator engagement also influences the educator. Wilcox and Lawson (2018) found that educators who scored high on engagement scales demonstrated higher levels of efficacy and emotional resilience when it came to facing the demands of system-wide organizational change. Put another way, they were less likely to burn out when faced with challenges at work. Karahan (2018) found that, when teachers achieved their goals, they were more likely to maintain engagement and be fulfilled at work. Educator engagement leads to more successful pedagogical outcomes and goal achievement and higher levels of personal career satisfaction and work wellness (Anikin, Lapteva, Kormin, Bondarovskaya, & Poletaeva, 2017).

To engaged educators, success is much more than mastering and sharing professional knowledge and skills; success in part is about positive social and emotional relationships with learners (Anikin et al., 2017). Positive educator-learner relationships, based on appropriate sharing and connection, can lead to "inner emancipation from the constraints of an increasingly cold system where success is too often based solely on performance metrics" (Kresin-Price, 2013). In our view, success as an exemplary educator—one who is genuinely able to say, "I love my work!"—stems from feeling engaged with learners and enjoying the positive connections within the educator-learner relationship. When educators believe that they provide high-quality teaching, and make strong connections with learners, they are also usually well satisfied with their careers. They can feel professionally fulfilled when their interactions with learners allow them to think that they made a difference for those individuals. Essentially, the experience of engaging with their learners can make the difference that fuels educators to continue to do their work in an exemplary way.

Likewise, from learners' perspectives, when participants in a learning experience (whether it involves attending a brief orientation session to learn about a new piece of equipment or enrolling in a course leading to a professional credential) believe that their educators care about them as individuals, their experience is likely to be positive. Positive educator-learner relationships have motivational effects on both parties. As Beaton (2017, p. 82) wrote, "just as students thrive in a safe, engaging learning environment, so do teachers." Such an environment is created, at least in part, by healthy and meaningful connections among all those involved in the learning experience (educator-learner and learner-learner connections).

But how can you as an educator continue the positive cycle of connection and net all the benefits that this sequence spins off, especially benefits such as staying motivated and enthusiastic in your educator role? How can you become the best you can be and avoid the burnout and rust-out that harm both you and your learners? Human connections have positive impacts on educators and learners. How can you as an educator facilitate successful connections with learners in which you get feedback that you have made a positive difference, for their benefit and your own career fulfillment, career longevity, and personal wellness? As a way of remaining in touch with times when your engagement made a difference to your learners, the strategy below is an invitation to reflect on special memories.

A STRATEGY TO TRY

Special Memories

At the beginning of this chapter, we shared a story about a special memory. The story described an educator who made a difference in the life of a learner. Although the educator did not fully realize how important the connection to the learner was during the learning experience, it became clear later. In this instance, the learner communicated in writing how much it meant to have a motivated and engaged educator remain present and available during devastating life events. Both the educator and the learner treasured the special memory.

Learners can communicate that they value relationships with their educators in different ways. Reflect on times when learners communicated that you made a difference. It might be an instance when a learner's face lit up with joy as you guided that person toward mastering a new skill. It might be an outpouring of relief when you granted an extension on an assignment due date. It might be a flood of tears when you took the time to listen.

These special memories are all stories of how your engagement with learners made a special difference, to them and to you. Is there a way to keep these memories fresh? During times when motivation seems to slip, how can you bring these special memories back into focus?

CONNECTIONS THAT COUNT

Many of you might recall a question on the admission form for your professional program: "Why do you want to be a . . . (nurse, or dentist, or respiratory tech, or physiotherapist)?" This question follows us throughout our careers. Then, as the work years go by, and some days are painfully challenging, the question changes slightly as you begin to ask yourself "Why did I *ever* become a . . . (nurse, or dentist, or respiratory tech, or physiotherapist)?"

In our view, unless educators can find ways to initiate and maintain positive connections with learners, those who feel as though they make a difference, they are at risk of succumbing to career killers such as burnout and rust-out. When educators function only as robotic teachers, making these effective connections becomes more challenging or perhaps even impossible. As the epigraph to this chapter notes, "robots are not people. . . . They have no soul." We would add that robots also have *no instincts, no warmth, and no compassion.* Robotic teachers cannot (at least at this point in the evolution of robots) make the same meaningful connections with learners that motivated and inspired educators can. We suggest three approaches that educators in any setting can implement to initiate connections and make them count.

First, attend to the little things; second, affirm the value of learners; third, share humour appropriately.

Attend to the Little Things

As Johnson (2019) quipped, "the difference between ordinary and extraordinary is that little extra." This applies to many aspects of professional success, including the education of health professionals. Attending to the little things is a simple approach that educators can employ to initiate meaningful connections with learners. When people connect and engage in any relationship, they notice the little things: actions, gestures, facial expressions, tone of voice, dress, pace of speech, attentive (or inattentive) posture, and deportment. We make judgments based on our experience of these elements, such as whether the person is interested in our opinions, cares about our experiences, or understands our perspectives.

In educational environments, invitational theory (Purkey & Novak, 2015) is foundational to understanding why some of these little things help to create and support connections among educators and learners. Invitational theory purports that successful educators invite (or "summon cordially") learners to participate actively in the learning milieu (Purkey & Novak, 2015, p. 1). Implicit in this invitational stance "is an ethical process involving continuous interactions among and between human beings" (Purkey & Novak, 2015, p. 1). Maintaining the humanity of participants in educational experiences, for both educators and learners, is essential to establishing and preserving connections. These positive connections help to maintain educator motivation, inhibit rust-out and burnout, and likely enhance the experience for learners.

Creating invitational learning environments that attend to the little things fosters human connections in both in-person and online settings. The process can seem to be more straightforward in traditional situations in which pre-service or in-service learners gather in a physical space. In online interactions, however, the little things still influence the possibility of a positive connection. For example, in online teaching, a quick response from an educator can indicate interest in the perspective shared by a learner, whereas a delayed reply (or no reply) from the educator can indicate a lack of interest in the comment or that it is not valued.

Tone is equally important in relationship building. Since online communicators do not have the opportunity to augment their messages with congruent non-verbal messages, tone can be more easily misinterpreted in the virtual world. Choosing precise words that relay the tone intended is essential to make the intended meanings of messages clear. When a visual component is included in online interactions through video conferencing, dress and deportment become essential elements. Just as in a university lecture hall or staff development classroom, so too in a video chat an unkempt look and messy background are clues to learners that educators do not value the interaction enough to look their best.

As we discussed in an earlier chapter, spending time on introductions at the beginning of a learning experience is important. In in-person settings, consider having learners form partnerships and introduce one another. In online settings, try having learners provide video introductions of themselves. Notice the little things that help to shape the connections within the group, either in a positive or in a negative way. In group discussions, identify commonalities and shared interests on which participants comment. Offer a personal response to each learner's introduction. Comment on something specific that the learner said, and ask a question to further the introduction as a way of humanizing the activity. As educators and learners get to know one another, the foundation is laid for the sense of class community and meaningful relationships.

After participants have introduced themselves, follow-up activities can help to make connections count. In in-person settings, allocate time for learners to locate (and do a small activity with) another learner in the room who shares a commonality. In online settings, invite learners to find someone else in the class (based on that person's introduction) to discuss a specific course-related question provided by the educator. These activities provide opportunities for each person in the course or workshop to work with (and get to know) another participant in a more meaningful way.

In 1965, Karl Rahner published a book called *Everyday Things*. It is a reflection on the daily round of common, ordinary things, everyday activities of living that we often take for granted. Facilitating introductions in any learning experience becomes an ordinary (expected and perhaps loathed) activity. By tweaking this activity to create more meaningful interactions, and by giving introductions the importance that they deserve, educators can use them to humanize the classroom and lay a foundation for a growing sense of community.

In addition to introductions, there are many other little things that skilled educators can do to forge strong human connections. To illustrate, we share a comment made by an educator in the health professions who teaches in an online setting. She commented on how nurturing the little things skilfully and with sensitivity engaged learners and left her feeling satisfied and fulfilled.

> I feel I have done my job well, and I feel most satisfied, when I make a strong connection with at least one student in a course. I try to keep notes on details about each student that they share during their introductions (and in their other posts). I start a spreadsheet with their name, location, where they are in their program, and details about their families, pets, etc. Very early in the first week I send each student a personal email where I reference something unique about them. For example, I might respond "Lilly it is great to have a student in the class with a special interest in. . . . We will be depending on you to add [to this topic during] our discussions. This will be invaluable." Inevitably I get a response back, and a conversation and fledgling relationship begin that can be built upon as the term continues.

This example shows a small educator-initiated action that takes little time but can lead to both enhanced learner engagement and, ultimately, educator career fulfillment. In the next strategy, we suggest how educators and learners can use artifacts that have meaning to them as a way of creating connections.

A STRATEGY TO TRY

Artifacts of Hope

Ask learners to bring (if you teach face-to-face) or share a photo (if you teach online) of an artifact that gives them hope. They then share with the class why this item is infused with hope for them. Educators also share artifacts and statements related to their hopes. In our teaching practice, some items that educators and learners have used include photos of inspiring people in their lives, a religious item, a picture of a child, and a package of flower seeds. As a variation of this activity, participants in the learning group can be asked to share an artifact that represents another human value or theme, such as compassion, honesty, courage, et cetera. This sharing of an artifact is a safe way for individuals to divulge their personas to the group, and doing so is foundational to creating connections.

Affirm the Value of Learners

Actions that affirm the value of others strengthen human connections and help people to feel satisfied and fulfilled. As we have emphasized throughout this chapter, experiences of satisfaction and fulfillment leave little room for burnout, rust-out, and low educator motivation. Educators, through their actions and words, communicate to learners that, no matter how challenging the learning journey becomes, they are available to support them in their learning. Educators let learners know from their first interactions that they value them as individuals and believe in their ability to accomplish their learning goals. Learners often enter educator-learner relationships in a more vulnerable position (at least they might perceive a power differential), and skilled educators find ways to minimize this perception and affirm learners' potential.

Educators affirm the value that they see in learners by finding ways to build upon their existing knowledge and skills. Opening learning activities with self-assessment exercises on a topic provides both educators and learners with an analysis of areas where learners are strong and where they need to develop further. Simply engaging each student in discussions (either in person on online using video) about a topic can help an educator to understand the learner's background knowledge. Once educators have a preliminary understanding of what learners know, they can involve them in peer-teaching opportunities in which they share their wisdom with other members of the learning group. Acknowledging and having learners share their knowledge comprise an overt demonstration of valuing.

Individualizing teaching approaches can also communicate that each learner within a group is valued. Courses and workshops designed (and taught) to maximize opportunities for learners to focus on their own priority learning goals and outcomes put them at the centre. Sometimes, to achieve this, educators need to be innovative and flexible, such as by providing a choice of learning activities and resources, so that learners can customize their experiences. Educators can personalize learning by supporting learners' individual goals and their voices and choices. When educators feel as though they are working within preset and rigid curricula, it can even take the bending or breaking of long-held approaches to individualize teaching approaches in ways that genuinely affirm the value of learners. However, the benefits for learners (and for educators) can make challenging the tradition or system worthwhile.

Successful educators believe in learners. They make every effort to see the potential in all of their learners and follow up with strategies that help them to realize their potential. In many instances, educators must remain creative as learners face challenges and struggle with progress. It might take some experimenting with various approaches to be able to connect with and consistently affirm that a learner is valuable. This is especially evident when learners have complex personal lives or have had limited academic success in the past. The following story demonstrates such a situation.

Helen was from a small town and had several children and an equal number of failed relationships that she disclosed to the class in the introduction forum of an online class. She had been working as a licensed practical nurse for 10 years and had not been in a formal learning situation since graduation. Now she was taking her first course online toward a baccalaureate in nursing. Helen also disclosed her self-doubt and fear of failure in her course introduction post. Her teacher noted this history and reached out to Helen with an individual email the day that she shared her introduction. In her email, the teacher congratulated Helen for taking this important first step toward her learning goal, acknowledged her feelings, and offered her support and encouragement. Then the teacher followed up with regular contact with Helen during the term, inquiring about how she was doing and reiterating her willingness to answer questions about the course or just to talk. At one crisis point during the term, Helen asked for a 24-hour extension on an assignment, which the teacher approved without question. Another time the teacher noticed that Helen had a special interest in patients with cerebral palsy (based on an example that Helen provided in an assignment), so the teacher located an interesting article on the topic and shared it with her. When Helen created an engaging video on the health issues faced by homeless people for one class assignment, the teacher asked her for permission to share her work with the class.

Helen passed the course and in an email to the teacher at the end of the course wrote "thank you for believing in my potential when I didn't believe in myself. You made all the difference." The notion of valuing learners can be summed up in the following poem:

Seeing the Shine
Every pebble
No matter how chipped and broken

Potentially contains
A dusting of gold.
(Perry, 2009)

An affirmation strategy follows. It can be used by peer learners or educators to enhance the sense of worth for class participants.

A STRATEGY TO TRY

Affirming Learner Creativity

It can be effective to have learners affirm one another. For example, if you and your learners value creativity in learning, then encourage them to notice when a member of the learning group has been especially creative. Suggest that they send a "warm fuzzy" text or email to that peer specifically outlining what they noticed. In in-person settings, learners can write a message about the person's actions and put them as anonymous notes of encouragement in a jar or other container to be shared at an appropriate time. Peer affirmation can be powerful.

Share Humour Appropriately

Shared humour and lighthearted interactions among people serve a social purpose that can facilitate the human-to-human connection. Karri, an exemplary educator, explained the social purpose of humour: "When you laugh with others, it tells them that you want to share something of yourself with them; and you get to know another part of them too. This gives a sense of solidarity. It creates a relationship that facilitates the work you do."

Humour in education goes beyond joking, clowning, and cartooning. Educators who effectively use humour to create connections with learners project a joyful attitude and zest for life. Educators who use humour well go beyond being a stand-up comedian or an entertainer; they convey a positive attitude or optimism and see the funny aspects of their worlds. Importantly, they open up opportunities for learners to do the same.

Astedt-Kurki and Liukkonen (1994) defined humour as *joie de vivre*, manifested in human interactions in the form of fun, jocularity, and laughter. They acknowledged that humour is a complex cognitive and emotional process. Hunt (1993) established that humour can be "many things to many people," that it must be interpreted, and that it is "whatever people think is funny" (p. 34). Classic humourist Baughman (1974, p. 54) identified humour as our sixth sense, as important as any of the other five:

> Much more should be said and written about humour, for so many think it means no more than the ability to tell a funny story or to respond to one. Actually, a sense of humour refers to a complete philosophy of life. It includes taking life's responsibilities seriously but oneself not too seriously. Other less obvious components of humour are these: the ability to relax, to escape from tension, to get pleasure out of the joys of others, to live unself-ishly, laughing with people.

This broad definition of humour is congruent with the attitude that motivated and engaged educators use to create connections that count with learners.

Humour and laughter are parts of sharing the lighter side of life, but this attitude goes further. It is an all-encompassing disposition, an ability to see the lighter sides of situations and encounters as they occur. It is a daily, moment-by-moment alertness to the possibility of seeing the funny, the humorous, and the laughable. This spirit of lightness serves as a lens through which educators can view their worlds and help others to see their own worlds differently. Fundamentally, an attitude of humour and laughter is incompatible with the experiences of burnout, rust-out, and low educator motivation that we discuss throughout this chapter.

Sharing humour or lightheartedness appropriately in any educational experience can be challenging. In in-person environments, in settings of both higher education and professional development, educators must always remain mindful of their professional presentation and learner sensitivities. There is always the possibility of misinterpretation (especially with attempts at humour). Timing is important since something that might seem to be funny at a time when a learning group is getting to know one another might lose its amusement during a time of stress, such as when learners are required to pass a test. The same is true in online environments. When communication is text based, the visual cues and tones of voice that can help learners to interpret an educator's intended meaning are absent. In an online milieu, the audience might be less known to the educator and peers, making it more difficult to judge what might be appropriate or inappropriate for that group.

When educators use humour and lightheartedness appropriately, there are several benefits. The first benefit is that communication among participants can be enhanced. Leacock concluded "but most of all, we laugh" (1938, p. 5). Educators who demonstrate a sense of humour also convey messages of openness and positivity to learners. Learners can view an educator who sees the positive in things, laughs easily, and smiles a lot as the kind of person with whom they are willing to share their learning goals and personal challenges. A smile, real or virtual, unlocks the doors to honest and meaningful exchanges. Being open to humour conveys that you are friendly, human, real, and approachable, the kind of person whom one can trust. Humour has an unmasking quality that allows for more personal and in-depth communication.

The second benefit of humour in education is that it promotes social presence, which occurs when members of a learning group project their individual personalities and develop interpersonal relationships with one another. Sharing lighter moments is part of creating a bond between educators and learners and among learners. When you spend time with others laughing and joking, it tells them that you want to share something of yourself with them, and you get to know another part of them too. This makes you friends in a way. It gives you a sense of solidarity.

Dean and Major (2008) support this belief as they emphasize that humour helps to establish relationships. The value of humour resides not in its capacity to alter physical reality but in its capacity for affective or psychological change that enhances the humanity of an experience. In particular, they point to the value of humour for teamwork, emotional management, and maintenance of human connections. You are acknowledging a person when you laugh appropriately. You are saying "yes, I understand what you are saying." Baughman (1974) describes humour as a "social lubricant." It eases social situations and promotes smooth and comfortable social interactions. Humour helps to establish relationships, decrease fears, encourage trust, increase friendship, and decrease social distance as it invites others to come close.

A third benefit of a lighthearted attitude is psychological. Humour itself is one of the good things of life, and it can ease tension in relationships and create moments of positivity. Humour provides a change of pace, injecting energy and optimism into the learning environment. A lighthearted attitude helps to relieve anxiety and tension. It is a positive outlet for frustration and lightens the heaviness of problematic situations. Humour is a tonic that invigorates, making an online class less drab and much more human. Gruner says of the psychological value of humour that "human societies treasure laughter and whatever can produce it. Without laughter, everyday living becomes drab and lifeless; life would seem hardly human at all without it" (1978, p. 1). As Archibald writes, "humour in the class room is like spice in the food—very necessary and important to add flavor and create interest" (2017, p. 118). Granato (2018) concludes that humour facilitates learning and challenges online teachers to take a risk and use "humour pedagogy."

Technology provides us with access to humorous content on almost any topic. In online settings, Archibald (2017) suggests, have learners submit a clip or funny cartoon relevant to a course topic. In in-person settings, educators can invite learners to share lighthearted items. Asking them to respond to peer submissions in a lighthearted way (or demonstrating it yourself) can perpetuate positivity.

Educators who move out of their comfort zones and use humour model a way for learners to add humour to their interactions as well. When educators inject positive words and funny examples into their lectures, presentations, commentaries, and online posts (or even if they smile or have a colourful background for their videos), doing so lets learners know that they appreciate humour and lightness, and it gives learners permission to respond in kind.

Amusing stories are also teaching tools that can help learners to apply theory to practice. Stories often help learners to achieve both cognitive domain and affective domain learning outcomes as they appeal to the emotions related to a topic. If the story has a funny angle, then it can be especially memorable and bring humour to the learning environment. Movies are essentially long stories, and they can provide powerful support for learning activities. Similarly, YouTube is a rich source of amusing short videos. Educators and learners can locate, share, and discuss them in most learning experiences. When learners have enjoyed and appreciated the inclusion of amusing stories in their learning experiences, they might be inclined to add a dash of humour or fun to their assignments or projects, furthering the goal of learning with positivity.

Sharing humour appropriately in educational experiences can nurture human connections. It does not need to take excessive time or effort by the educator. As we mentioned, it might require educators and learners alike to move out of their comfort zones and embrace new challenges. In doing so, educators can develop a greater repertoire of teaching strategies and gain a sense of satisfaction and fulfillment. Humour is not a skill that robots possess; it is a human action and interaction. In the following strategy, we share insights from psychologist Maurice Elias (2015), who encourages educators to begin a process of cultivating humour by laughing at themselves.

A STRATEGY TO TRY

Humour Starts with You

According to Elias (2015), everyone benefits when humour is part of the pedagogy since it builds learning relationships "through the joyful confluence of head and heart." You are not trained as a stand-up comedian or entertainer; sharing humour and creating a class in which humour is cultivated and appreciated for its positive effects on learning start with educators who laugh at themselves and the things that they say and do. When you make a slip of the tongue, put something in the wrong place, call a learner by an incorrect name, forget what you were going to say, laugh at yourself. Poke fun at your flaws and foibles. Doing so sets an example for learners and lets them know that they can also take themselves a little less seriously and that it is acceptable to have fun while learning. Shared humour reduces tension in the classroom, helps students to improve retention of information, and sets the tone for a positive emotional experience that they share with each other and their teacher.

CONCLUSION

This chapter encompasses ways of thinking and approaches that educators might appreciate when feelings of low motivation, rust-out, and even burnout emerge. We shared ideas that provide insight into maintaining motivation. Engagement can make the difference between an excellent educator and a robotic teacher. As we have emphasized throughout this book, the human connections are what count. Attending to the little things, affirming the value of learners, and sharing humour appropriately are just a few of the many ways in which educators can connect with learners.

In Askinazi's (2004) words, "connection is a gift" in human relationships, and it can be transcendent for educators and learners. When they connect in meaningful ways, a cyclical process of positive, joyful invigoration can develop. This circle of transcendence can be a powerful motivator and reminder to educators everywhere about why they chose to teach. We close with a poem by Perry (2009) that attempts to capture, within the limitation of words, how transcendent the essential human connections that we have written about throughout this book can be for all people in a relationship.

The Circle of Transcendence
Sometimes as a teacher,
when I think about
the vastness and complexity of the world,
I am overwhelmed.
I feel so unimportant,
so insignificant,
so powerless.

Then,
I meet you,
and by creating a small connection,
I make you feel valued.

The result is a wonder.
When you feel important,
so do I.

It is so simple.
It is so profound.

REFERENCES

Alpaslan, G., Bozgeyikli H., & Avci, A. (2017). Sinif ogretmeni adaylarinin basari yonelimleri ile mesleki kaygi duzeylerinin incelenmesi [An investigation of primary school pre-service teachers' achievement goal orientations and occupational concerns]. *Journal of Abant Izzet Baysal University Faculty of Education, 17*(1), 189-211

Alvandi, M., Mehrdad, A. G., & Karimi, L. (2015). The relationship between Iranian EFL teachers' critical thinking skills, their EQ and their students' engagement in the task. Theory and Practice in Language Studies, 5(3), 555.

Anikin, I., Lapteva, S., Kormin, A., Bondarovskaya, L., & Poletaeva, O. (2017). Pedagogical conditions for highly productive activity for teachers of higher education establishment. Journal of Entrepreneurship Education, 20(3), 1–8.

Archibald, C. (2017). Reflection: Lessons learned from teaching online in undergraduate programs. ABNF Journal, 28(4), 114–118.

Askinazi, A. (2004). Caring about caring. Nursing Forum, 39(2), 33–34.

Astedt-Kurki, P., & Liukkonen, A. (1994). Humor in nursing. Journal of Advanced Nursing, 20(1), 183–191.

Baughman, M. (1974). Baughman's handbook of humor in education. West Nyack, NY: Parker.

Beaton, A. M. (2017). Designing a community of shared learning. Educational Leadership, 74(8), 78–82.

Bridgeman, P. J., Bridgeman, M. B., & Barone, J. (2018). Burnout syndrome among healthcare professionals. American Journal of Health-System Pharmacy, 75(3), 147–152. doi:10.2146/ajhp170460

Broeckelman-Post, M. A., Tacconelli, A., Guzmán, J., Rios, M., Calero, B., & Latif, F. (2016). Teacher misbehavior and its effects on student interest and engagement. Communication Education, 65(2), 204–212.

Brown, M. (2015). Rust-out: The unfamiliar cousin of burn-out! Retrieved from https://www.sixthsenseconsulting.co.uk/rust-out-the-unfamiliar-cousin-of-burn-out

Čapek, K. (1926). Rossum's universal robots. London: Penguin.

Clouston, T. A. (2015). Challenging stress, burnout and rust-out: Finding balance in busy lives. London, UK: Jessica Kingsley.

Cowin, L. S., & Moroney, R. (2018). Modelling job support, job fit, job role and job satisfaction for school of nursing sessional academic staff. BMC Nursing, 17(1). doi:10.1186/s12912-018-0290-2

Dall'Ora, C., Ball, J., Reinius, M., & Griffiths, P. (2020). Burnout in nursing: A theoretical review. Human Resources for Health, 18, 41. doi.org/10.1186/s12960-020-00469-9

Dean, R., & Major, J. (2008). The relational humor inventory: Functions of humor in close relationships. Journal of Clinical Nursing, 17(8), 1088–1095.

Edelwich, J., & Brodsky, A. (1980). Burn-out: Stages of disillusionment in the helping professions. New York, NY: Human Sciences Press.

Elias, M. (2015). Using humor in the classroom [Web log post]. Retrieved from https://www.edutopia.org/blog/using-humor-in-the-classroom-maurice-elias

Garrison, D. R., Anderson, T., & Archer, W. (2000). Critical inquiry in a text-based environment: Computer conferencing in higher education model. *The Internet and Higher Education, 2*(2–3), 87–105.

Granato, J. T. (2018). *How do faculty at the University of New Mexico use humor in online teaching?* Doctoral dissertation, University of New Mexico, Albuquerque, New Mexico, US. Retrieved from .https://digitalrepository.unm.edu/oils_etds/40

Gruner, C. (1978). *Understanding laughter: The workings of wit and humor.* Chicago, IL: Nelson-Hall.

Hunt, A. (1993). Humor as a nursing intervention. *Cancer Nursing, 16*(1), 34–39.

Johnson, J. (2019). The difference between ordinary and extraordinary is that little extra. *Good reads.* Retrieved from https://www.goodreads.com/quotes/254906-the-difference-between-ordinary-and-extraordinary-is-that-little-extra

Karahan, B. Ü. (2018). Examining the relationship between the achievement goals and teacher engagement of Turkish teachers. *Journal of Education and Training Studies, 6*(3), 101–107.

Kresin-Price, N. (2013, January 1). Building warmth sculpture in the student-teacher relationship: Goethean observation and contemplative practice in an action research inquiry. ProQuest LLC.

Leacock, S. (1938). *Humour and humanity: An introduction to the study of humour.* New York, NY: Henry Holt.

Leider, R., & Buchholz, S. (1995). The rust-out syndrome. *Training & Development, 49*(3), 7–9.

Maslach, C., Schaufeli, W., & Leiter, M. (2001). Job burnout. *Annual Review Psychology, 52*, 397–422.

Milburn-Shaw, H., & Walker, D. (2017). The politics of student engagement. *Politics, 37*(1), 52–66.

Perry, B. (2009). *More moments in time: Images of exemplary care.* Edmonton, AB: Athabasca University Press.

Purkey, W., & Novak, J. (2015). *An introduction to invitational theory.* Retrieved from https://www.invitationaleducation.net/docs/samples/art_intro_to_invitational_theory.pdf

Rahner, K. (1965). *Everyday things: Theological meditations.* London: Sheed and Ward

Riley, J. (2018). *The relationship between job satisfaction and overall wellness in counselor educators.* Doctoral dissertation, Capella University, Minneapolis, Minnesota, US. Retrieved from https://eric.ed.gov/?id=ED580552

Shirom, A. (1989). *Burnout in work organization.* New York, NY: Wiley.

Wilcox, K. C., & Lawson, H. A. (2018). Teachers' agency, efficacy, engagement, and emotional resilience during policy innovation implementation. *Journal of Educational Change, 2*, 181.

We extend our sincere thanks to Pamela Holway at Athabasca University Press for her wisdom, inspiration, and guidance throughout the process of creating this book.